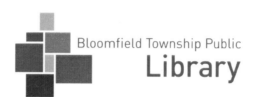

THE
YOGA
LIFESTYLE

Dedicated to Sara Hanoch
Beyond being a loving mother, you are an inspiration to many—
Living in wisdom, love, and adaptability—a true flexitarian.

DORON HANOCH

Foreword by Mark Stephens,
author of *Yoga Sequencing*

THE
YOGA
LIFESTYLE

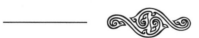

Using the Flexitarian Method to Ease Stress,
Find Balance and Create a Healthy Life

Llewellyn Publications
Woodbury, Minnesota

First Edition
First Printing, 2016

The meditative approaches in this book are not a substitute for psychotherapy or counseling nor are they a substitute for medical treatment. They are intended to provide clients with information about their inner workings that can add another helpful dimension to treatment with a trained medical or mental health professional, as their circumstances may warrant.

Book design by Bob Gaul
Cover design by Lisa Novak
Cover image by Erin Blair
Editing by Gabrielle Rose Simons
Interior art by Germán García Fernández

Llewellyn Publications is a registered trademark of Llewellyn Worldwide Ltd.

Library of Congress Cataloging-in-Publication Data
Names: Hanoch, Doron, 1971– author.
Title: The yoga lifestyle : using the flexitarian method to ease stress, find
    balance & create a healthy life / Doron Hanoch.
Description: First edition. | Woodbury, Minnesota : Llewellyn Publications,
    2016. | Includes bibliographical references.
Identifiers: LCCN 2016002999 (print) | LCCN 2016009926 (ebook) | ISBN
    9780738748665 | ISBN 9780738750521 ()
Subjects: LCSH: Hatha yoga. | Medicine, Ayurvedic. | Vegetarians. | Health. |
    Stress management.
Classification: LCC RA781.7 .H363 2016 (print) | LCC RA781.7 (ebook) | DDC
    613.7/046—dc23
LC record available at http://lccn.loc.gov/2016002999

Llewellyn Publications
A Division of Llewellyn Worldwide Ltd.
2143 Wooddale Drive
Woodbury, MN 55125-2989
www.llewellyn.com

Printed in the United States of America

Disclaimer

The content and information offered in this book is not offered as medical advice or medical opinion, and is not intended to treat, diagnose, prevent, mitigate, or prescribe the use of any technique as treatment to any illness or disease, nor to any physically or emotional problems.

This book is not intended as a substitute for advice from your physician or health care professional. You should consult with a health care professional before starting any new diet, exercise, breath work, psychological, or supplementation program, or if you suspect you might have a health problem.

Any health advice in this book is intended for information only. Any review or testimonial offered in this book does not guarantee any type of outcome. They are anecdotes and do not serve as scientific research.

Contents

PART I: THE BASICS

Chapter 5: Breath Work—

PART 3: WORKING WITH THE PROGRAM

Chapter 8: The Flexitarian Method as a Yoga Lifestyle...325

Acknowledgments

I bow in deep gratitude to all my teachers along the way, including Osho, the Dalai Lama, Daido Roshi, Shugen Sensei, Pattabhi Jois, Mark Stephens, Richard Freeman, Tim Miller, Rolf and Marci, Vin Marti, Adarsh Williams, Chris Price, Sheshadri, BNS Iyengar and Cidananda, as well as my teachers at the Natural Gourmet Institute. There were many more formal teachers as well as informal, beautiful beings that were happy to share their wisdom with me over a cup of chai in India, a glass of wine in New York, a meal at Esalen, or while breaking bread in one of the many countries I've been fortunate to visit.

Thank you, Erica Goewey, for the first round of editing of this book, your friendship and your wisdom.

Thank you, Maria Kuzmiak, for being a master editor and sharing your amazing insights and eye for detail.

Thank you, Mom, for believing in me and encouraging me to stay true to myself, and thank you, Gil Hanoch, for the support throughout this book creation process.

Thank you, Lauren Anas, for all your help and support, and to all of my students for practicing, for asking questions, and for allowing me to share with you the wisdom of the ancient and the modern teachings that support each one of us on the way to liberation.

Lastly, thank you, the reader of this book, for taking the steps to learn and grow, for your willingness to embark on this beautiful journey that will hopefully not only bring you bliss and joy, but will also allow you to spread it on.

Foreword

In practicing yoga, we gradually come to discover that it affects the entirety of our lives. How we eat, sleep, think, and feel all take on new qualities. Our lives get better as we come to know ourselves better and better through the mirror of practice. The deeper we go with it all, the more we come to appreciate the joyful and transformational nature of yoga. For some, this inspires a deepening sense of caring about others and the world, which inspires a desire to share the practice with others.

When I met Doron Hanoch in my classes nearly ten years ago, it was clear from the beginning that I was in the presence of a man deeply devoted to his practice. Yet as serious as he was (and is) about yoga, he was equally light about it, always finding simple and humorous ways to explain what it's all about. His genuine humility was all the more meaningful because of the depth and commitment of his practice—a practice that extends well off his mat and into every aspect of his life.

Along with his passion and insight for all things yogic, Doron is a masterful chef who appreciates the beauty of food as an essential nutrient for the soul, as well as for a healthy body and mind. He's also a consummate citizen of the world, whose extensive travels are reflected in his very broad yet deep appreciation of diverse cultures and peoples. Add the wisdom that comes from daily practice and deep contemplation, and you find a man who is wonderfully gifted in teaching about yoga and thriving in this life.

We are now blessed to have Doron's experiences and insights into what he sensibly calls a flexitarian life, brought together in his new book, *The Yoga Lifestyle*. Sometimes it seems that there are many various disconnected ideas, concepts, and practices in the yoga realm. Doron makes the connections clear, revealing how one might best cultivate the balances in life that make every breath, every bite, and every moment altogether more sublime.

Mark Stephens
Author of *Teaching Yoga*, *Yoga Adjustments*, and *Yoga Sequencing*

Introduction

There is a plethora of meditation, yoga, health, nutrition, and cookbooks on the market. Many of them address a specific diet or dogma, in which they treat the person as if we all have the exact same body and mind. One can argue that in essence we are all the same, but on a functioning level, we sure are different.

This book describes a holistic system to accomplish a yogic lifestyle within the modern world. Traditional concepts of yoga are explained in clear, contemporary terminology. You will find Sanskrit names with English translations. The book offers a toolbox of the most efficient practices that may fit into today's lifestyle, mining tradition to create powerful contemporary practices. Kept simple, the book provides foundations without an overwhelming amount of unnecessary detail, and provides essentials that can be utilized right away in life.

The Yoga Lifestyle introduces the concept of the flexitarian. If you've heard the term, it's probably with respect to the flexitarian diet, which most people define as a diet that is mostly vegetarian or vegan but does include some fish, poultry, and meat on occasion. The book looks at the flexitarian diet and expands upon those principles to create an entire flexitarian lifestyle. *The Yoga Lifestyle* aims to create the best life possible, without the stress. It seeks the healthiest life options for each individual, according to his or her needs.

Is This Book for You?

Have you ever wanted to:

- Understand yoga and learn how to build your own practice?
- Know your body type and balance your life?

- Live in sustainable health and happiness?
- Be empowered with practical and efficient tools for a healthy lifestyle?
- Develop a steady and focused mind?
- Become stronger and toned, without lifting weights?
- Become flexible, without being a ballerina?

The Yoga Lifestyle is great for anyone willing to take responsibility for his or her own life. It is based on the research of many yoga traditions (mostly from the ashtanga vinyasa tradition), mind and meditation practices (mostly Buddhist and Gestalt), as well as most health diets, both modern and traditional (Ayurveda, blood type, macrobiotic, raw food). It takes the best from each dogma and presents a system that each person can adapt to meet his or her individual needs.

Health, a Holistic Matter of Body and Mind

When I sat down to write this book, I first thought to focus on just yoga poses. I love the practice and it made a great positive change in my life. What I noticed was that my practice was very influenced by what I ate the night before, and even my overall diet influenced my practice. Certain foods created mucus and stiffness, while others helped lubricate my joints and helped me be alert and limber.

Then I thought of food; I love food and what a great way to tap into one's overall health. You are what you eat, or more accurately you are what you digest. But in order to digest well, you need to have a body that works well. To improve digestion, we can massage the internal organs with some yoga and practice some breath work. We can also keep a stress-free mind, to improve digestion and assimilation of nutrients.

I can't really teach yoga without tapping into food. And yoga already incorporates breath work and mind work into its practices. A graceful, healthy, sustainable yoga practice can only be done with a healthy body and a healthy mind. Without the mind in the right space, it is hard to achieve a positive outcome. A healthy mind is really the foundation for creating a life of bliss.

When people ask me what my secret for staying healthy, fit, and happy is, I tell them that it is about keeping life in balance, taking a holistic approach—this is the modern yogi—flexible enough beyond the body to adapt to the needs and changes of the world we live in today.

If I had focused only on one element (physical yoga, breathing, food and nutrition, or mind work), my life would have improved for sure, yet I would have still suffered until I worked on all levels. You can have a great engine in the car, but if your wheels are completely worn out, you cannot expect the car to run well and safely. Even if the engine and wheels are both in great shape, if the windshield is dirty, you will not be able to see where you are driving.

It is not about choosing one thing to work on; it is about incorporating all of the elements that we need as humans to experience a healthy lifestyle: an active and supple body; breath for balanced energy; healthy, wholesome food in moderation; and a sound mind that makes conscious decisions that are good for you and the environment, now and in the long run.

You may have ups and downs—welcome to being human! The holistic approach to health helps you ride the downs with a smile, or at least without the great suffering that may come from them. You will be empowered to take action to move from the downs back to a balanced state of being—a state where you can enjoy the highs and deal with the lows without agony.

I hope to inspire you to take steps on all levels of your life. The modern yogi—you—is a flexitarian that incorporates yoga into all layers of her life. This will transform your work, your relationships, and your surroundings. You will become like a radiating light, illuminating all that comes in contact with you.

Finding balance takes time. It starts with small steps and being consistent. You do not need to be "good" at yoga to start practicing it. You do not need to be at the "right weight" to have a healthy diet. Practice the methods offered in this book regularly and you will have a sustainable, joyful life. So how can you maintain holistic joy?

The most important step is to keep your life balanced and avoid extremes. By doing this, you don't need to keep readjusting and fixing things. Though you may be living in balance, keep working on all aspects of your health throughout the day, every day. Maintenance is the key to a sustainable yoga lifestyle. This means *The Yoga Lifestyle* is going to walk with you throughout life.

While thinking is helpful, it is also important to give your mind a break. We will learn how to do it later in the book. The answers to holistic joy will unfold as we go through the chapters, and learn to use the four-part system of the yoga lifestyle.

The Flexitarian Method

"Are you a vegetarian?" I am often asked. "A flexitarian," I answer.

A what?

Well, I could say I'm a "healthatarian," a "blissfultarian," or a "joyfultarian," but I've decided on flexitarian, because this describes my attitude of always acting with mindfulness but not adhering to rigid discipline.

My mission statement is simple: Live a healthy, active, and joyful life; maintain balanced energy with breath; eat good, nutritious food; practice mindfulness; and celebrate life while minimizing stress and negative effects for yourself and your surroundings.

How Is This Done?

Choices are made in the best way, according to each situation. This means that you have to practice awareness with all that you do. Some people have no problem being vegan, and feel great with it. Other people may find that small amounts of eggs or even fish work better with their lifestyle, blood type, or just overall health. We all have different constitutions, and at different times, we have different needs.

When buying food, seek the best ingredients you can afford. Organic vegetables are a priority. Fruit comes next. Include some raw food as well as fermented food in every main meal. If buying animal products, then again, try to buy the best quality and the most humanely-raised animals—grass fed, free range, and organic. If eating out, choose what will make you happy for the moment but will also allow you to feel good later in the day, or the next morning on the yoga mat.

Will you have another drink? It is easy to say yes without thinking, but it's important to really check and see how you feel now—and to be honest with yourself about how you will feel later. At times, this means you may decide to go home and eat your own home cooking or even eat something before you go out, so you only consume small amounts of foods that do not truly serve you. When visiting others, try to make the best choices, but just like when traveling, if there is something new that you would not ordinarily eat because it's not the healthiest option, you may decide to give it a try. Keeping an open mind is a key principle of being a flexitarian. *The most important element of the flexitarian lifestyle is awareness! Every decision is made with awareness and not out of conditioning.*

The goal of the flexitarian is to be happy and content. It is not about following any one dogma, any one religion, or a guru. There cannot be any one diet, any one yoga sequence that will suit us all the time, let alone suit all beings, all the time. We each have different needs and these needs change constantly.

The flexitarian invests some time in creating a toolbox. This is what *The Yoga Lifestyle* is for. Educate yourself, so that you can make the best choices possible for each moment, while understanding that change is inevitable and thus the learning experience is ongoing, as well. With the new toolbox, you will grow empowered and learn to carve your own way, discovering the sculpture within.

Main Elements of the Flexitarian

1. **Be happy**—The goal of our being is to live in joy and share it with others.

2. **Do not harm**—We seek joy with as little negative impact as possible on others, the planet, or ourselves.

3. **See the big picture**—Life is more than just your ego. When you are willing to surrender into the greater energy, nothing is lacking.

4. **Be a whole person**—In all that you do, consider the mind and spirit, as well as the physical body. Each part of us is fully a part of the whole; ignoring one part will surely lead to dis-ease.

5. **Stay balanced**—Overall balance is a priority over temporary excitement. Maintain the balance from the roots up, from the basics.

6. **Flow with nature**—Allow the wisdom of nature and the universe to guide you. Listen to it, and follow the path of least resistance.

7. **Listen to your gut feelings**—You know the answers, you just need to pay attention to the signs and the wisdom that is beyond the thinking mind.

8. **Listen to your body**—It also has answers. Even answers to emotional problems are apparent, when you are fully aware of the symptoms in the body.

9. **Prevent illness and suffering**—Take action now to improve yourself on all levels, including being better to others, and you will prevent illness and suffering in the world.

10. **Empower yourself**—Take responsibility for your life; your actions, words, and thoughts create your future.

PART 1

The Basics

Any architect knows that a good building needs good foundations. If you set up your basics well, you will find it much easier later to keep the practice going in a sustainable manner. Many people decide to improve their lives—pick up a sport or a new diet—but unless there are some supporting tools in place, they tend to drop the practice.

We will set our goals here, and learn how to keep getting closer to them with small intentions. We will learn about general lifestyle practices that will help us clean, inside and out. Laying good foundations first allows you to progress much faster later.

In this first part you will also learn the basic tendencies you have and may not be aware of. Ayurveda will be introduced, and more specifically the dosha system that will help you know what the right practices are for you, and how to practice them.

The Ayurveda section will give a great deal of information in a short time. Not only will you know much more about yourself, but you will also know what to do in order to come back to balance and stay in balance. Though this section is for you, I have had many students who used this information to learn how to live better with other family members, partners, coworkers, and spouses.

The basics are good for this book in its entirety, but are good stand-alone foundations, as well. These basics can be applied to any other practices you may have, as they are general and empowering when you know how to apply them in your life—as it is now, or as a yoga lifestyle.

— 1 —

The System

Before we go any further, take a moment to thank yourself for taking the time to read this book, even if it was given to you as a gift. You are reading these lines, so you have already taken the first step. If you just continue one step at a time, a life of bliss will become an ordinary part of who you are—you will be a modern yogi. The modern yogi does not seek to escape ordinary life, but rather integrate yoga into it. She simply lives her life in a holistic healthy manner, practicing the four elements of this book—physical yoga, breath and energy, food and nutrition, and mind training.

This is your first step toward a life of unconditional joy. At first, some of the information might seem overwhelming or to require too much effort, yet soon enough you will realize how effortless a life of joy can be. It is like riding a bicycle. At first, it is intimidating and difficult to find the balance, but you know that it will be great once you can ride smoothly. You try, and maybe fall a few times, and then get the hang of it. Before you know it, you just get on the bike and ride, enjoying the fresh air and the motion. You don't really need to focus on the process anymore. It is the same with creating a yoga lifestyle. Go through these steps, start practicing, and you will find that the practices become super joyful and easy, and the effects on your life become transformational. So let's leave the suffering behind and step together toward a life of joy, the life of a modern yogi!

The Process

Let's roll out the plan and see where we are heading.

First, we will set our goals and intentions, and next, we will present some foundations, creating the healthy lifestyle principles and attitudes that will help us with all the practices we will do later.

Once we have our basic set of lifestyle practices, we will take the next step and learn a bit more about ourselves. Using the tools of Ayurveda (the dosha system), we will learn how to evaluate where we are in our life, at the moment. We will learn how to identify what is out of balance and the causes of imbalance, and we will learn practices to get back into balance.

Then we will look at the tools that will help us gain health and happiness. We will begin with yoga, learning the different poses and how to practice them. Then we will learn about breathing techniques, followed by the food chapter where we will get some basic understanding of how to make good food choices. Finally, we will learn about the mind and techniques for training it, including a variety of meditation techniques.

Though I present the yoga section first, it is important to read and begin the mind practices as well as the food and diet practices as soon as you are comfortable with them—hopefully all at the same time—so reading through the entire book first can be extremely valuable to get an overview. Then you can look at the practice manuals in Part 2 to get ideas about how to incorporate this information into a practical practice.

In some yoga traditions, one has to master the *asanas*—the poses—before going on to *pranayama*, or breath and energy work. Only after mastering asana and pranayama would one continue on to concentration and meditation. The idea is that it is easier to work with our body than with our mind. In this book, we are not going to choose one over the other; indeed, the bodywork will be a great part of our initial practice, but the mind will be an underlying tool, the one setting the tone. We will use the physical practices to get healthier in our bodies, as well as to train our minds. I use a holistic approach to work on all aspects simultaneously, yet you may find that you focus more on one element to begin with, and that is fine. However, it is important that you notice if you are skipping some practices altogether, and to understand why you are doing so. Sometimes we avoid what we need most to grow. There is no need to force anything, but with a playful attitude, we will try to build a total sustainable life.

Along with the physical practices and mind practices, we will start to look at what goes into our bodies. We will essentially learn to be our own doctors and cultivate the ability to listen to our body and identify what it needs. Food and nutrition go hand in hand. Once we know the ingredients that serve us well, and understand the basic effects they have on how we live, it will be easier to create our diet.

Review of the Process

- Read through the entire book and begin with some of the simple practices in the book as you go.

- Develop a deeper practice in all areas, by continuous practice.

- It may seem hard at times, but be patient and don't give up!

Find the middle path, a place where you are happy to show up to practice and can practice with joy—a place where you progress safely and enjoy the process. This is the best way to move more quickly toward your goals in a sustainable way.

Setting a Goal—the Destination

What is your final goal? Why did you buy this book? What are you looking to change, achieve, or grow into? There may be things in your life right now that prevent you from feeling completely joyful. Not everything can be changed, but a lot can—especially YOU! So let's think in terms of YOU. What is YOUR goal?

Achieve your goals only if you *know* what your goals are. This step is one of the hardest to take. You don't need to know exactly or specifically what it is that you are in search of, but many of us do have an idea of some things that we would like to change. It might be as simple as being happy, more relaxed, losing the stress, the weight. Perhaps you have a more complex goal in mind, like finding out who you really are: a simple question with an answer that can only be discovered by you.

My Story

I grew up in Israel and was told that I am Jewish. It even said so on my identity card, yet I always wondered what it meant. Could I choose my religion? If so, why was it decided for me? Who gave me this identity called Jewish or Israeli? Why did they not consult with me first?

As a toddler, I spent three years in Texas. I had an Israeli background now mixed with some American conditioning. This was the first step of shaping my international thinking. I visited Europe with my parents for a month when I was twelve, with many trips to small villages and mom-and-pop bed and breakfasts. At thirteen, for my bar mitzvah, I was given the option to visit New York and New Jersey with my younger brother instead of having a big party—the norm for a bar mitzvah celebration. Of course I took the trip to the USA. I was the guardian of my eleven-year-old brother, and we stayed with American families, some religious and some not. During our stay, we discovered break dancing, Bruce Springsteen, a video game arcade, and many things I did not know about growing up in Jerusalem in the '70s and early '80s. It was 1984. Who was I then? An Israeli? A wannabe American?

Later, during my three-year compulsory military service, I felt more confused than ever about who I was; I couldn't find the meaning of life and was starting to feel very depressed. I could not comprehend why people were fighting, why they were so close-minded regarding their views, and why they were willing to risk their lives for these views.

I felt happy with some of the simple things I had, but was not sure what I was supposed to achieve in life, what my purpose was. I would go from one extreme to another. One day it seemed to me that I was supposed to be a millionaire by the age of thirty. Some days I felt I was born to be a spiritual leader, while on other days, I was contemplating methods of suicide. Because I did not know what happens after death, I did not have the courage to kill myself.

I needed answers. As I finally finished my military service, I embarked on a journey to Asia, a very common journey among young Israelis, yet my journey was different. I left on my own, just my backpack and me. I told my mom I'd return in two months or two years. She was supportive.

I was on a quest—the search for a reason to live and an understanding of who I was. It seemed to me that we go through life running after our tail, trying to get somewhere, but the only place we all reach is death. My journey took me to many spiritual teachers and centers. Every center I entered, every teaching I heard, every yoga practice I did, and every form of meditation I practiced never really directly addressed my question, but somehow gave me a non-logical reason to keep practicing, to keep finding out the truth for myself.

It was seeing the great masters and how they lived life and handled situations, hearing their words and seeing their actions that drew me closer to understanding what I wanted. I wanted to achieve their state of mind, their vitality and the radiant joy that projected from them.

The first time I entered a Zen monastery, I just knew I needed to be there. I was immersed in feelings of clarity, simplicity, and security.

The pursuit for understanding health and happiness has continued throughout my life. While running my art and photography studio in New York City, I practiced Tibetan Buddhism and Zen. I practiced a variety of yoga styles, learned from each one, but committed to the ashtanga vinyasa, Mysore style. I loved the self-practice aspect of it, but not that the practice was the same every day. This is why I developed my own system, so you can do a self-practice, but still have variety in your sequences.

Within the realms of food and nutrition, I experimented with a variety of diets, from vegan to raw food, from macrobiotic to vegetarian. Since none of them worked for me all the time, I eventually became a flexitarian.

Beyond formally going through a holistic cooking school and studying nutrition, I kept on reading and researching these topics with vigor, and with continuous study and experimentation. I worked with family, friends, and clients to keep refining the best practices for health and happiness. Over time I realized that there is no one answer to all, which is where the flexitarian method was born.

I took all the traditional tools I learned and merged them into my Western life. I became a modern yogi—living a yoga lifestyle while still continuing with the ordinary life. A yogi is someone who practices yoga on all levels: physical yoga, including breath work, eating well, and having a healthy mind. A yogi is someone that cares about themselves as well as the environment and others. Some claim that the female version of yogi is a yogini. For simplicity we will use the term yogi for both male and female.

What Do You Need?

To find the peace and joy that I found, you do not need to travel to Asia or join a Zen center, though sometimes stepping out of your element helps. Some people go on a yoga retreat to step away from their everyday life and give themselves time to reflect on what it is that really matters.

Since this book focuses on health and happiness, what matters to you? What do you need in life to be happier and more fulfilled? Do you know? Is it confusing? Maybe you have many ideas. Consider putting it all down on paper. Be as detailed as you can. Write down everything that comes up. Don't try to edit or make it pretty, just write; this is only for you. Ask yourself: What do I need? What do I really want as an ultimate goal? If you could design your perfect self (most joyful, healthy self, etc.), how would you like to be?

Now read it.

Stop and read it again. Feel it in your gut. How does it feel? Read it out loud. What resonates as true? What jumps out? Is it something specific or something more abstract, like *be happy*?

Now sit down, close your eyes, and try to envision yourself in the state in which you want to be. What do you look like? How does it feel? Pay attention to every detail and make it become real in your mind. What are the obstacles that prevent you from being in that state?

Now that you know where you are going, you can put your goal aside. It will be there always, and you should be able to keep seeing yourself in that state, but do not get attached to any timetable.

Review: Setting Your Goal

- Sit down comfortably and quietly with your spine tall, not leaning.
- Ask yourself: What do I really want? Then, write it down. Let it flow without editing.
- Visualize yourself in your ideal state and feel it in your body; try to embody and be what you really want.
- Write down the obstacles that are preventing you from getting there.
  Then again, try to come back to your ideal state and let it really sink in.

Setting Intentions—Short-Term Goals

Having a goal or destination is important, but once we know what it is, we need to work toward it with mini goals—or intentions—that are short term and easier to manifest. Setting intentions is part of the process of reaching your goal. If, for example, my goal is to realize enlightenment, I can't just close my eyes and have it. Well, technically I can, but for most of us it doesn't work that way. It is like saying my goal is to be healthy, fit, strong, and free of illness. Wonderful. Since we can't just blink and make it happen, we need stepping stones to take us across the river to our destination. These stepping stones are little steps toward your goal that you can achieve within a limited timeframe. These are your intentions.

An intention may be something that will keep you in balance or help get you into balance. For example, if you have a stressful day ahead, commit to taking two deep breaths every thirty minutes, and before you make any important decision. Maybe your intention is to eat a healthier lunch or to meditate for ten minutes every day. These are tasks that you know you can do. You may want to skip them, make up excuses for why you can't do them today, or why you don't have time, but setting an intention is like signing a contract. It's a commitment. So set intentions that you know you will actually do. You can set grandiose goals that may seem romantically beautiful, but it's more important to be realistic and set intentions that are somewhat challenging, yet still within your reach. I'm not saying you should find excuses for not following through; rather, enjoy setting intentions that do take you further—that encourage you to practice and improve. Set goals for a relatively short amount of time—a daily intention, a weekly intention, and maybe a monthly intention. You can always extend your intention over and over again.

Every morning as you wake up, have a ritual of setting your daily intention and connecting with your weekly intention. Maybe the weekly intention is set every Sunday night or Friday morning—whatever works for you; just be consistent. Decide on a time of day to set your intention, say in the morning after washing up and before breakfast. Sit down, look at your watch, and give yourself five minutes. Maybe set a timer, so you know you have a full five minutes just to sit and reflect. If you decide on your intention in one minute, spend the rest of the five minutes visualizing yourself in that state or manifesting your intention. It may feel silly, and you may feel that you already know your intention, but at least for the first month, make sure you give yourself these five minutes daily. Treat it like a spiritual ceremony. Do it with enthusiasm. This is where you start manifesting your dream.

Tips for Setting Your Short-Term Goals

- Wake up and wash up. Be effective and mindful.
- Set the timer for five minutes and take your seat.
- Visualize your goal. See it clearly. Then remind yourself of your weekly mini goal.
- Check in. How do you feel? Set your intention for the day according to what you feel you may need today.
- Envision yourself practicing your goal. See it as clearly as possible.
- When the five minutes are over, give yourself a smile of gratitude, knowing you are actually going to do this.

Commitment—The First Step: Show Up!

So you know where you want to go and you have even been able to set up smaller daily intentions, but maybe you've already found that after two days, you seem to slack. *I am running late today, feeling tired; oh, I'll just start again tomorrow.*

Setting up a routine—a ritual of practice—is as important as any part of mind training. This is true even if you know exactly what your intention will be or you think that having a routine is useless; that is your mind taking control of you. Remember, we are looking to take control of the mind.

So maybe your first intention is to simply show up. If you don't show up, how will you practice? How will you make any improvement? This is why we start with setting intentions for goals that we can actually meet and build up from there. When you have a feeling of success—of achievement—you *will* take the next step because you will be encouraged to keep going. Even small achievements give the mind the stimulation to keep going. But the slightest disappointment will cause the mind to create excuses—why now is not the right time, or why this practice may not be right for you, or you are not the type for this, and on and on. The mind is very creative; let's keep moving forward positively. For now, your intention may simply be to read through this entire chapter by the end of today or tomorrow. No step is too small.

Taking a small step at a time is always a good idea, especially when challenges arrive. For some, the food will be the most challenging aspect of improvement; for others, it will be the meditation or the movement. It really doesn't matter where the challenge is as long as you are committed and make these constant small steps toward improving. Show up to do the work, no matter how insignificant it may seem.

So if your intention is that of commitment to the practice, work on just showing up for five minutes each day to set your intention. Even if you end up fiddling and daydreaming for the whole five minutes, your mind and body will get used to getting up and preparing, and most importantly, you will eventually set up new standards of commitment.

To help you stay connected to your practice, create rituals to help you realize your goals. You may decide that before meditation, you will light a candle or refresh the flowers. Maybe before you do yoga, you will light incense or simply look at an inspiring photo of a yoga pose and say, "Thank you for the inspiration." Sometimes having a small, fun, and easy ritual is the first step toward developing a longer practice. I love to start with a few breaths, feeling my body and offering gratitude for the opportunity to practice.

On days that I don't feel like doing a yoga practice, I simply show up and do small things that I love. I watch my fingers take out a match from the box, the movement of the match as it strikes the box, and the magic of the flame that appears. Slowly, I light a candle. Candles make me happy. Then I sit at the top of my mat and take a few breaths, feeling gratitude expand from my heart. I slowly move onto all fours for some cat-cow (see yoga section) to release the back. Maybe the next step will be to just try a low lunge. I keep going slowly, until, like an old engine, something clicks and starts running. Then I keep going with my practice. But the first step, no matter how much I didn't feel like it, was to show up. Something always happens after that, but without showing up, nothing will happen.

Show up, do one small good thing, then another. Before you know it, your life will transform into a holistic practice.

Show Up! How to Make Your Practice Happen

- Create a ritual—something you look forward to.
- Do something, even if it is just showing up and standing on your yoga mat with your hands together at your heart. Then see what happens.
- Incorporate rituals into all aspects of your life. For example, practice gratitude before a meal, light a candle before meditation, chant before yoga practice, or bow in gratitude to the shower before you use it.
- Consider making a chart to track your progress each month. Then, every day after you set your intention, mark a checkmark next to that day or post a fun sticker.
- Congratulate yourself for showing up. Tell yourself, "Just one more little thing…" Then go for it. At the same time, don't worry too much about the future. Live in the moment.

Do the Best You Can in Every Situation

If you can show up, smile, and do your best, you're headed in the right direction. Really, you can't do more than that anyway. Well…at times you can; you may want to push yourself harder on an exercise day or during a yoga practice, but that is not always for the best. When we push too hard, we can burn out or get injured; injuries force us to slow down much more than if we would go slowly to begin with. I used to like to push hard because I wanted to get over the hard work part and be flexible or strong or enlightened. I did see quicker progress but also got injured at times.

When I was injured, my mind would come to "save" me. Now I had excuses for why I couldn't practice, which allowed me to step out of the race, a race my mind had invented. This way I felt my ego was protected all the time. When working hard, I seemed to be strong, and when injured, I could say it was due to the great work I had done. This way of living worked at first but quickly became old. I was not really happy to be injured, and when I needed to get back to the practice, it was torture. I was out of shape. I had fallen off the wagon, and it was hard to pick up again.

Life can get a bit too intense when we constantly try too hard. Even if we do feel that we are progressing due to hard work, we will almost always move faster and with greater ease if we learn how to practice with grace and compassion. Do the best that you can, without judgment or great expectations. This does not mean you lose sight of your goal or intention; it just means you do your best to get there and are okay with whatever the outcome is. As you will see, not all days are the same. Some days you will wake up with a clear mind or an open body, and then the next day may be different. At any given moment, if you simply do the best you can and enjoy where you are at the moment, you will begin to experience the joy of practice as well as the joy of life. Then you will be more likely to stick with the practice and see results.

How to Improve Happily and Efficiently

- Do the best you can without judgment or expectation.
- Accept where you are today and enjoy it.
- Don't be hard on yourself.
- Practice with grace and compassion.
- Remember that going slower can sometimes get you there faster.

Standing on the Shoulders of Our Teachers

This principle of a new artist practicing in the arts is true for anything: First you study and receive teachings, and the more you practice, live, and breathe these teachings, the more you embody what you've learned, until you create a specific set of spices for your own recipe, so to speak.

"Practice and all is coming," claims Pattabhi Jois, the father of ashtanga vinyasa yoga. It is not by talking about yoga that one becomes a yogi. Indeed, reading and discussing is important, but it is the practice in everyday life that creates an artist, a teacher, or a master. This practice is what then allows the master to embody the teachings in an authentic way.

Ganga White, a prominent yoga teacher who studied with many masters, tells us that we should be "standing on the shoulders of the past" (White, 2007). In other words, we need to respect the ancient and previous knowledge, and then take it a step further.

An artist, a yoga teacher, a musician, or even a philosopher starts with studying masters of the past. Practicing yoga and studying with great masters is of great value. At a certain point, after substantial practice and time, you may find this knowledge engrained within you. Once the knowledge is there, you may begin exploring what works for you, what feels right for you as an individual. This is the point when you have acquired a great toolbox of knowledge and possible practices, and you can decide which of them will become your own and how you can modify them to really fit who you are. At this stage, you become your own master. Don't rush to this stage. Take your time to practice with teachers, and always keep practicing and studying. There are moments when the ego feels it already knows everything. Make sure to question your ego regularly.

The tradition, the teachers of past and present, are guides—shepherds presenting the grass. Once we can see the grass, we can try to eat it and see if the teachings resonate with us. Then give it another bite; at first it may be bitter—new—but eventually, we may learn to see the benefits. Maybe with the guide of a wise one, we may learn how to chew, how to digest, and how to use the new powers we gain.

The teachers that I respect the most are those that empowered me, not controlled me— those that were sharing all they had without holding back. They were willing to show me all there is and accept me for who I am.

I hope this book will empower you in the same way and allow for these teachings and practices to merge with your current life—incorporating the yoga lifestyle into your life. I intend to share with you all that I know and all that worked for me, including tools that I have created from my own research and practice, either new or a mix of highlights of the best information I gathered from different sources—my own salad of practices.

Really living in joy—having a blissful life—is something that will be truly yours only through your own experience. You can learn about many things and even recite what you learned, but it is only when you actually live it through experience that you attain mastery.

I have learned a great deal from my teachers and masters, but it is through my own practice—my own experience and my own realizations—that I have come to be who I am. I hope that you, too, will use this book as a guide and as an inspiration to practice so that you may live your life in a new and fulfilling way with ownership of your life and your happiness.

Practices for the Ultimate Student

- Study diligently, and practice what you study.
- Have respect for your teachers but stay authentic.
- Master the basics before you dive into the advanced.
- Be okay with always being a student—even when you become a master.
- Give gratitude towards your teachers daily.
- Eventually be okay with finding your own path.

— 2 —

Laying Foundations:
Lifestyle Practices

Life goes on far beyond the sixty-minute yoga class, or twenty-minute meditation. We know we want to practice sustainable health and happiness by including the four elements of the flexitarian method, but in order to sustain the practice, we need to set up some healthy lifestyle habits—from staying clean to good sleep. Following these steps will ensure we are prepared for the four element practices that we will practice later.

Empower Yourself/Your Teachers and You

Asking questions is fundamental to any kind of growth. We have a few ways in which we learn what is true for us:

1. From our own experiences;

2. From what other people that we value have told us;

3. From accepted standards, such as the law of physics.

All three ways can help us understand reality, but we must realize that each one of these on its own is usually not good enough to make us sure about the answers we seek. It is important to listen to other people's advice, opinions, and teachings, though it is equally important to learn to question these teachings. The first step, however, is to trust the teachings of teachers you respect, and practice these to gain your own personal experience. Then question and verify if they work for you, so that no matter how big the name of a teacher, and no matter how many other people use this information or follow this method, you will be able to keep checking for yourself if the information holds true.

Learning from peers and from others, as well as from others' experiences, is a fantastic tool, but you really must learn to have confidence in whatever you are experiencing and in your interpretation of the teachings. This is true, of course, for everything in this book, as well. I write here as a teacher, shining the way with my understandings, interpretations, and experiences of a very wide variety of practices, from many other teachers. Not many people can afford the time, effort, and money that I have put into studying and practicing these modalities, and so this book tries to create a toolbox of the most efficient practices I have found and used to create a blissful life.

Many times we follow what society dictates for us as truth. We come to believe that the norm is the right way, without really stopping to question it. I lived in Italy for a while, where it was a custom to break for an espresso and a smoke often. I joined in, as it would have been weird to go do yoga in that setting. I learned later to surround myself with people whose norms and standards I actually appreciate, so that they inspire me to do better. Some norms or social standards were created during a certain era when they were needed, but they are no longer appropriate for today. Other standards were created for certain societies or different generations, and are not relevant to you as an individual. However, it is important to look at social standards and notice their benefits, because many times they do have a teaching to offer us, and there is no need to rebel just for the sake of rebellion.

The important thing is to make conscious decisions about every action, so that we are not moving on a path that does not belong to us. This is more than just the saying "follow your truth" or "be yourself." Conscious decision making is absolutely essential in order to find your bliss. By living according to your own truth, which may be based on respected teachings, you will be able to go to sleep feeling absolutely wonderful and sure that whatever decisions you made today, even if they were wrong, were *your* decisions made with a clear mind.

This is true for any and all dogmas. A dogma isn't necessarily inherently wrong, or doesn't have substantial goodness to offer. It is just important to remember not to follow anything blindly. If you find dogma in a teacher that really does resonate, then it is important to trust that teacher, even if at times it might seem not exactly what you would expect. And still within this following, you must keep a questioning mind, so that if the requirements of the teacher or of the dogma do not sit with you anymore, you are fully aware and can be responsible for taking care of yourself.

Even though there are great masters out there worth following—and trusting, true masters will accept questioning students—though they may encourage you to trust the process or method, it is up to you to discern when to follow and when it does not feel right for you anymore.

There is absolutely great importance in having a teacher, someone who can help you with the process that you—specifically you—are going through. The teachings might be coherent, but the way that you, as a student, receive them will never be the same as the way another student receives them. This is true for anything from meditation to nutrition to yoga asana practice. Hopefully, your teacher will become an important part of your support system. If you have more than one teacher that you work with as you are finding your bliss, do try to limit the number of teachers you work with, so that you do not get confused by too many systems. And, it is also helpful for a teacher to see you regularly, so he or she can get to know you better and be able to guide you through the process.

Teachers in many cultures are revered with the highest esteem, as they are the ones that have the most capability to empower you and help you discover what you really need. Paying respect to the teacher in any way possible is important, but at the same time, you have to join in as a partner with your teacher, and do actual work yourself if you really want to see results. Reading and philosophy are very good, yet unless you convert philosophies into practices, they will remain ideas and not living truth.

Review of Your Teachers and You

- Find teachers you respect, and practice what they teach for a while.
- Check in to see if the teachings resonate with you.
- Make sure you are not running ahead because of impatience or unwillingness to do the work. Be happy to take the teachings and eventually carve your own path.
- Continue to respect your teachers, even if you have found a way to mix your own salad of practices. It is through their teachings that you discover your own way. Learn to listen clearly to what is true for you and follow it.

Sustainable Living

Living sustainably means living without hurting our surroundings or ourselves. In regard to food and the earth, a sustainable life will protect future generations on this planet. For the purposes of this book, let's focus on how we can live more sustainably today, in order to maintain health and joy in a balanced manner.

First, let's see how we can maintain our practice for the long run. As discussed earlier, if you push yourself too hard today, you may get injured and not practice for a month after. In other words, pushing yourself will not be sustainable. If you sit in meditation for so long that you become miserable and decide to never try it again, that is not sustainable. You may decide that you enjoy your long sit, especially after a long asana practice, but because you devoted so many hours to your practice today, you will be running after your tail to catch up with life over the next few days. That may not be sustainable either.

You want to find a practice that you can maintain as a normal routine that will be strong enough to allow progress, and also feel great so that you will be encouraged to come back and practice again. The same goes for eating and everything else we do in life. If you go on an extreme diet, it is more likely that when you come off of it, you will be feeling deprived and gorge on food. There goes all the hard work.

A good diet is a diet for life, a diet that becomes a part of your healthy lifestyle, one that is sustainable because it is easy and pleasurable to maintain. While some people can go running while maintaining ease, for many of us it is better to go on a feel-good walk than a stressful run. Work slowly toward building up endurance and love for the things in life that are better for you; it's important not to burn out too quickly.

One of the most dangerous ways many of us push ourselves is in our jobs, usually in our attempts to make money. Do you ever find yourself so overworked that you just keep making mistakes? Do you ever fall asleep at your computer, or start to doze as you're driving home from work? Do you work so much that you become ill and need a few days to recover? Knowing how to live a balanced life is important on all levels.

Not all of us suffer from overworking. Some of us are plagued by the opposite traits: lethargy, idleness, or laziness. For so many reasons, many of us have a difficult time getting motivated to do anything that requires real work. We may find ourselves in debt, out of a job, or just miserable with what we do. We may neglect our bodies until they are in such bad shape that we don't even know where to start. Putting off our duties—whether in work, in relationships, or toward ourselves—can leave us so overwhelmed that we can't even begin to consider getting back on track. No extreme is good or sustainable.

Acting today in consideration of tomorrow, doing what we can today within our means of body, mind, and abilities, is the way to a sustainable life.

Sustainability Tips

- Make wise decisions; everything you do will have a future effect.
- Find moderation.
- Do something that is good for you every day, even if it is small.
- Keep the momentum when you do find yourself meeting your goals.
- Increase your practices gradually.
- Respect where you are, and start making small breakthroughs.
- Take one step at a time, but DO take a step!
- Enjoy the present, but remember that it affects your tomorrow.

Take Away Distractions and Hurdles

When I was a chocoholic, I could not resist eating a whole chocolate bar once I opened it. It was the same when I shifted my addiction to ice cream. Before I could come to my now very-easily-controlled quantities of sweets, I had to simply not have them available. If I was at home and I did not have chocolate, I did not eat it. If it was there, I did. So I started by taking away this distraction and temptation from being too readily available. When your willpower is not as strong as you would like it to be, don't try to challenge it!

Some of the things we may be addicted to are fine in small doses but are not good for us in excess. Since it is not easy to simply decrease the amount of whatever it may be we do too much of (eating, watching TV, sex, smoking, drinking alcohol, etc.), we may need to take stronger measures for a while, to help reduce temptation. You may decide to clean out all the sweets from your home, hide the cable of the TV (or place a blanket over it), encourage drinking buddies to engage in healthy activities with you, or avoid going to certain places where you know the temptation will just be too strong. Over time—once the addiction isn't controlling your life as much—you may reintroduce some of these things back into your life consciously, with awareness and moderation.

Learn to say no. It is sometimes easier to please friends or people and say yes to foods, activities, or actions you don't really want to consume or be part of. Why do you do this? Many of our actions come from habits or past conditioning. It may be that as a child you wanted to please your parents, so that they would let you stay up late to watch a show, or give you a treat or money. Now this habit transforms and pushes you to please other people for the wrong reasons. Find the source of the habit, recognize it, and then practice acting differently instead. This is the practice of reconditioning.

Sometimes it is easier to simply remove the distraction or source of addiction from our lives, and other times we need to plant a new seed—a new habit—to replace the old one. For example, if you are used to wanting a treat in the afternoon, and you are used to opening a specific cupboard because that is where you store your sweets or your potato chips, try replacing this food with healthy snacks. The healthy snacks should occupy the same place as the less healthy treats, because you already know it's the snack place; now, however, when you open that cupboard, you will find kale chips or nuts. Maybe make fruit very visible in a beautiful bowl near the cabinet—or a smiley sign that says, "Fruit is in the fridge. Yum!"

If your distraction is on your computer—an announcement or a program, for example—keep it closed and don't go there every time you get an alert. When I was writing this book, I would constantly be distracted by announcements of incoming email or Skype messages. I decided to close all the programs I was not using at the time, and only open them after a few hours of work. This helped me focus and kept me on track. I used to pride myself on being a multitasker, until my Zen teacher said this to me one day: "What is it with people running with music in their ears? When running, run; when listening to music, listen to music." Be completely present with what you are doing.

What are your distractions? It may be that you need to turn off your phone for periods of time, silence it, or take an app break. We all have different weaknesses, things we do on auto-mode and not with full awareness. The easiest way to avoid them is to simply stay away from them for a bit, and in the meantime practice awareness of all that you do in the moment (or strive toward it), so you are conscious of what you are actually doing at any given time. This is not like running away from something or stopping a behavior forever; it is more like a cleanse—a system to stop you from automatic habits and conditioning—that will lead you toward a life of acting with awareness.

Review of Distraction Cleansing

- Before any task, stop, take a big breath, then go and do it.

- Only answer the phone when necessary (and after a deep breath).

- Keep your phone on silent when you need to focus, or when eating, or when you are with friends.

- Choose your friends and activities wisely, and learn to say NO.

- Keep sources of distraction and addiction away from easy reach.

- Do not bring home anything that is not great for you.

- Limit the number of tasks you do at once.

- Limit the number of open programs on your computer and use only the apps that you actually need.

- Practice awareness of all that you do.

Dissolving Judgment

One of the hardest things to do when starting a journey to better yourself is the practice of no judgment: not judging who you were, what you did, or how you are doing now. Self-judgment serves no purpose. Mostly it just occupies our head, and keeps us from moving forward.

This is not to say that we should be ignorant of the mistakes we have made. We learn from our past, but there is a difference between learning from the past and self-judging or being overly critical. The difference is mostly in the outcome. Your practice is to recognize what you have done, learn from the mistake, and then take actions that are beneficial, constructive, and empowering. Find motivation through self-encouragement, rather than self-judgment or abuse. For many of us, judging comes automatically, almost like an instinct. As soon as you recognize that you are judging, smile and just shift your awareness to see what can be done to make it different for the future. Like any habit, this too can be dissolved.

Judgment can happen toward others, as well. This can also be destructive, as judging others happens when you compare them to an ideal or to yourself: "He is more flexible than

I am. I cannot believe she just said that to me. Why would anyone wear such a hideous dress? Why does today's generation obsess about the Internet and their gadgets?" At times, it can become a whole story: "Why did he have to cut into the lane here? It's so dangerous, and now I need to slam on my brakes. If only everyone stayed in their own lane, it would all be so much better, but of course, he is driving a Jaguar. My uncle owns a Jaguar, and he would totally do this too. It's been a long time since I actually spoke with him. Maybe I should call."

This can go on and on, expending futile energy and wasting time. Take a deep breath and just let the person cut into the lane! Keep enjoying the music or simply stay focused on the road, making sure this distraction does not lead to a car accident.

Practice awareness of your mind, of the stories created there, and come back to the present moment time and time again. Make sure not to judge yourself for being judgmental! It sounds funny, but it can easily happen: "Oh no, I just made up a story again. Oh, I was still comparing myself to her all through class." Be compassionate toward yourself, and over time, the critical mind will soften as well.

Review of How to Dissolve Judgment

- Do the best that you can, and be okay with where you are now.
- Learn from the past and move on. Encourage yourself to keep going.
- Don't worry about how others are doing. Focus on what you can control.
- Be compassionate with yourself and others.
- Stay present!

On and Off the Mat (or Becoming a Saint)

The practice of yoga helps us find our authentic selves. Yoga practice is about personal growth and finding the ultimate freedom; it is about knowing your true self. The process involves everything we do in life, and goes beyond the specified practices of exercise and meditation. It is how we live our life in every moment, the choices we make, and the actions we take.

There may be many times in life when we take an action that may not be something we would be proud of, or believe is a good action, and most likely we will never be caught. Should we still do it? Maybe it is self-serving. Maybe it is just a habit. It can be anything from slumping in a café, eating certain foods, or not taking care of other people's possessions (such as a yoga mat in a studio).

If you find yourself doing anything that you feel a bit guilty about, or that makes you feel as if you need to check to see if anyone is watching you (because you do not want to be seen doing it), then this is something you probably should not do. This will save you worry and will keep you doing only what you know is the right thing to do, which ultimately lets you stay relaxed and happy.

I like to imagine that there are TV monitors everywhere, and what I do may be transmitted to all my students. Since walking the talk is very important to me, I try to make every decision as if all my students were watching. You can imagine that, at every moment, your actions and thoughts are being broadcast to all the people you value the most. Would you be doing this if your mother knew? How about your boss or wife? Saints are not special people. They are like you and me, except they are committed to doing the right thing from a selfless, heartfelt place.

Live a moral and sound life—a life that allows you to feel absolutely good about what you are doing at every moment. Don't choose this lifestyle because it is the right thing to do, but because you know deep inside that it is right. Everything can be twisted to suit your needs if you want it to be.

Make sure you really believe in what you are doing, knowing that as you say a word, think a thought, or take an action, you are behaving in a way that can lead to a better you and a better world.

Your behavior should be *at least* equal to what you expect from others. The way others conduct themselves should never become an excuse for the way you behave. Stay true to yourself, your standards, and beliefs, not in a dogmatic righteous way, but in a compassionate, loving, and kind manner.

Review of How to Maintain Goodness

- Practice being honest and good every moment of your life.
- Live your life as if, at every moment, the people whose opinions you value are watching you.

- Have no worry about being caught doing something wrong, because you don't do wrong.

- Be stress free by knowing you do what is good for you and others, so others will always be grateful to you.

The Power of a Smile

One day in class I asked my students to stretch their legs and arms, open their hips, do an extra *chaturanga* (low push up), and eventually to stretch their lips to their ears—yes, to smile while practicing a pose. They took all of my physical challenges with no hesitation, except for the smile. I had to ask them a few times until I had most of them actually moving their lips slightly.

I questioned them. "Why is it that if I ask you to do harder work, to stretch deeper or to do an extra chaturanga, most of you, no matter how hard the request and how much suffering is involved, will go for it immediately, though when I ask you to smile, very few actually do it?"

This happened in a very "go-getter" environment. Of course some people love to smile and smile often. If you do not smile often and for no reason, check and see—do you take yourself too seriously? Do you feel better doing things in life that are challenging, that may even induce some pain, but not doing one of the easiest and most rewarding actions of turning your lips up to smile? Do you feel guilty about being happy? Do you need a special occasion to smile? Is it socially awkward to just smile for no reason, or worse, while "working out"? It's not too late to change it!

A smile is easy and free. The very simple act of stretching the lips introduces relaxation and softness while releasing happy hormones in the body. Smile to your loved ones, to a flower, to a random person, and even just smile to yourself. No reason is needed.

Smile Practices
- Make smiling the first thing you do as you open your eyes.
- Anytime you feel a bit stressed, rushed, or anxious, take a big breath and smile.
- Smile at people you meet.

- Smile periodically throughout the day to allow happy hormones to be released in your body.
- Smile before you go to bed.

Sleep Hygiene or Tips for a Good Night's Sleep

On a summer family trip to the Sierra Mountains of Northern California, a long hiking day came to an end.

"Have a good nothing," my sister-in-law Debbie wished my brother Gil, and I wished him the same. "Have a good nothing," he replied.

"Now that my diet is so much better and I exercise more, sleep is my next issue. I tend to wake up at night and just go into thoughts, planning, or thinking of clients and their needs," my brother Gil had told me one day.

Meditation was the first suggestion I offered. Meditation (described in chapter 7) is simply training the mind. It is sitting still, doing nothing, allowing our awareness to drop to the belly as we follow the breath, in and out, in and out.

Take our legs, for instance. When we go to sleep, we want them to be still and resting. There is no need for them to move. The same goes for our eyes or ears, but what about our mind? Why is it so hard to just switch off the mind? A good night's sleep is a night of rest, a night where all functions of the body, except for the autonomic systems (like the heart or breath), are resting, including our digestive system and our mind.

Gil seemed to be okay with the idea of meditating and was willing to give it a try, though his first reply was, "It will be hard to fit into my schedule." Since his mind is a very strong one, and since he has the capability of making decisions and following through on them, he decided to convince his mind that there is no need for it to do anything during the night. It can all wait for the next day. Simply do nothing.

Indeed, doing nothing is the hardest thing for most people in today's fast-paced world. Yet doing nothing is really the ultimate rest. "This is your vacation time," Gil had to tell his mind before he went to bed. "A time to have a good nothing."

The next morning, Gil woke up with a smile. He was determined enough to control his mind into shutting down when it needed to, but for many of us, it is not that easy. We may need to practice convincing our mind that we do not need it to work during the night, that it is good for it to rest.

Since just telling the mind to stop thinking is not such an easy task, using the breath is a great tool. Lie down in bed and breathe slowly and deeply, fully bringing awareness to the breath. You may want to count your breath. Slow inhale—one—slow exhale—two—and so on until you reach ten. The slow rhythm of the breath and its calming effect helps bring about peace and surrender. If you have regular insomnia, consider practicing the one-to-two breathing described in the pranayama section as you lie in bed.

It helps if you go to sleep before 10:30 pm. According to Ayurveda, after 10:00 pm we begin a new cycle of energy. During this energetic cycle, we sometimes feel that we get a second wind. So if you are sleepy, go to sleep when you are sleepy. Otherwise, you may get that second wind and lose your sleep opportunity.

If you do not fall asleep within thirty minutes, get up and do something that will induce sleep and then return to bed. (Note: Some sleep specialists recommend you never leave the bed; in this case, have something really boring to read nearby. You need to decide what works best for you.)

Your mind has an easier time when it knows what is about to happen. Create a routine. Go to bed and wake up at the same time. This will keep your wandering mind in balance.

Exercising is healthy and useful for a good night's sleep, but timing is key. Finish your exercise at least three to four hours before bedtime. Mornings and early afternoons are the best times to exercise.

Eat dinner at least two to three hours before bed. If you are hungry later, have a light snack—a small piece of fruit or a few spoonfuls of unsweetened cereal with a bit of almond milk, or simply sip a small cup of hot chamomile tea.

Avoid caffeine, nicotine, and alcohol for five hours before bedtime. For some, this is less of an issue. Learn to notice your body after you have caffeine. It may seem like no big deal, but try and also notice your mind and speech. Do you think more, or faster? Maybe not so good before sleep.

Drink plenty of water during the day so you don't need to drink much at night; ideally, you should not need to get up for the toilet during your sleep time.

Make your bedroom a sanctuary. Use soft light, and keep it clean, inviting, quiet, and relaxing. Try to avoid having electronic devices in the room. If you do, keep them as far from you as possible, and maybe even cover them with a nice fabric. I had a TV in my room for a while, just to watch movies sometimes. Since I rarely used it, it had a nice Indian fabric covering it, giving a peaceful atmosphere.

Use your bed for sleeping and sex only. Read, work, watch TV, and fold laundry elsewhere. This way your body will recognize that being in bed means sleeping.

Take a hot bath an hour before bed. The drop in body temperature will make you feel sleepy, and it is nice to get into a clean bed with a clean body.

Develop bedtime routines. Listen to quiet music, sit silently, read something calming, or massage your body with oil. This is good for you in general. It helps you to relax, have a nice ending to your day, and it can help give a sense of closure to all the activities of the day. I notice that when I do this, I feel much better, especially since I don't feel anymore that my days are just blended one into the next.

Do not turn on lights during the night, even if you have to go to the bathroom. Exposure to light during the night impairs melatonin production, which is crucial for a good night's sleep.

Get some sunlight as soon as the sun is up, as it will help set your biological clock.

A good night's sleep is the secret to a happy and productive day. It is the time our body takes to restore and rejuvenate. Our night depends on the day we had, and the next day depends on how well our previous night was.

Sleep, like *savasana* (corpse pose) in yoga, is a place to have a good nothing—a place to surrender and just allow deep relaxation. So from now on, I wish you "a good nothing."

Review of Sleep Hygiene or Tips for a Good Night's Sleep

- Go to sleep when you feel sleepy.
- Create a routine. Go to bed and wake up at the same time. Go to bed before 10:30 pm.
- Finish your exercise at least three to four hours before bedtime.
- Make your bedroom a sanctuary, and use your bed for sleeping and sex only. Keep all electronics out of your bedroom while you are sleeping.
- Develop bedtime routines. Listen to quiet music, sit silently, read something calming, or massage your body with oil. Take a hot bath an hour before bed.

- Eat dinner at least two to three hours before bed. Drink plenty of water during the day, so you don't need to drink much at night, and avoid caffeine, nicotine, and alcohol for five hours before bedtime.

- Do not turn on lights during the night, even if you have to go to the bathroom.

- Get some sunlight as soon as the sun is up, as it will help set your biological clock.

If needed, as an extra measure:

- Take melatonin (2–3 mg thirty to forty-five minutes before bedtime) for a few weeks, and then let it go.

- Take magnesium (500 mg) thirty to forty-five minutes before bedtime.

- Sleep well and wake up smiling. Have a blissful life!

Cleanliness and Skin Care

This may seem obvious to some, but keeping a clean body, clean clothes, and clean surroundings is key to happiness and a healthy body. When cleaning anything, it should be done from a place of gratitude. I have never had a cleaning service for where I live. I do my cleaning a bit as a workout—cleaning mirrors like *Karate Kid*, scrubbing the bathtub, and wiping surfaces. I do it with passion and power. Some part of cleaning is meditative for me—vacuuming, dusting, washing dishes, and folding laundry. These activities offer me an opportunity to practice gratitude for all the things I use: the floor, carpet, sink, toilet, kitchen, and so on.

Even if you do have some of your cleaning taken care of by others, there will always be things you need to do yourself. Keeping everything clean and tidy regularly allows you to keep clean and organized in the mind. If you go to bed with a dirty sink, then that is what you will have to see in the morning. If you leave clothes on the floor, the next day you will wake up to a messy room. And for many this becomes a pattern, and the mess increases over time. As it increases in your outer world, so it may increase within your mind too. You do not need to become fanatic or germ phobic, but use common sense and keep things clean and in order on a regular basis.

Taking showers regularly, as well as using a cloth for scrubbing the skin at least once a week, is very important. After scrubbing the skin, make sure to moisturize it, ideally with oils. A combination of sesame and coconut will work for most people. You can also mix in almond oil, as well as your favorite essential oil (e.g., lavender, lemongrass) for scent if you like. Keep your hair, nails, and ears clean as well.

Here are two Ayurvedic practices I find useful:

Tongue Scraping

If you look at your tongue in the morning, you may find it has a white coating on it. This coating is bacteria, dead cells, fungi, and toxins that the body does not need, known in Ayurveda as *ama*. Cleaning the tongue in the morning is a good practice for aiding the body to rid itself of unnecessary toxins. The simple way to do it is to scrape some of it off, using your toothbrush after you brush your teeth. This is good, but the toothbrush is not made for a spongy surface, such as the tongue. There are tools made specifically for tongue scraping, which are inexpensive and more effective than the toothbrush. The common tool is a curvy piece of metal or plastic that is dragged from the rear of the tongue forward, to scrape off the toxins. This may help with bad breath as well as improving overall health and even refining your sense of taste. I highly recommend scraping the tongue every morning.

Oil Pulling

Since the mouth in general hosts lots of bacteria, it can be extremely beneficial to clean it. Scraping your tongue and brushing your teeth are important, but another practice you may consider is oil pulling. Oil pulling is a practice of swooshing oil around the mouth for twenty minutes so that the oil pulls out the unnecessary toxins with the saliva. You can use sesame or coconut oil for this. Personally, I prefer the taste of coconut oil. First thing in the morning, before you drink any liquids or eat any food, take a teaspoon of coconut oil and place it in your mouth. For me, half a teaspoon works just fine, as I produce a lot of saliva. The oil may be solid or liquid; either way is fine. It will dissolve soon enough. Swoosh it around for twenty minutes and then spit it out into the trashcan. Rinse with warm water that has a quarter teaspoon of baking soda dissolved in it. You can do this every morning while you shower, make your bed, or do light stretches.

Review of Cleanliness and Skin Care

- Clean up after you are done eating.

- Floss and brush your teeth regularly, scrape your tongue daily, and do oil pulling. Scrub your body/skin at least once each week.

- Oil your skin at least twice a week (more often if you have dry skin or there are heaters in your daily environment that dry your skin).

- Wash your hands with soap as needed, and avoid using antibacterial gels.

- Keep your surroundings neat and clean; put things away immediately after you finish using them.

- Clean one extra thing each day. For example, when you see the light switch is getting greasy and black, take a break from what you are doing and go take care of it.

- Use clean clothes, towels, and yoga mats.

— 3 —

Ayurveda:
Personalize Your Life!

We are all one, but we are not all the same. Neither are we the same every day, nor every season. We will understand later what it means to be all one—all part of the same thing—but first we will understand ourselves as individuals. When we know ourselves and are able to take care of ourselves, we will be better able to be whole as beings, and serve others with our goodness. Ayurveda is an ancient Indian method that was designed to bring people into balance. Ayurveda means "the science of life." When I was in the Natural Gourmet—a healthy cooking school—we learned a variety of health systems for diagnosing others and ourselves. When we used the Ayurvedic system, I found it to be the easiest way to understand where I was in terms of balance (body and mind). In this book, I will not offer the complete Ayurveda system for coming back to balance, but rather focus on the tools for understanding and assessing yourself, so that later you can use a variety of tools—including but not limited to Ayurveda—for healing and balancing your life.

Most systems that seek to improve our health look at all beings as if they are the same—with the same needs, bodies, and tendencies. These systems prescribe one diet or one exercise program to all. The founder has the answer, and it is the best answer, and thus we should follow. In many cases, a system like this is very suitable for the founder of the system, and some individuals will find it suitable as well. This does not mean that it works for everyone, all the time. Not only are we different beings with different bodies and tendencies, we also live in different climates, have different daily routines and professions, and have different types of food available to us.

The Dosha System, a Tool for Understanding Yourself

Since many diets and systems have great offerings, if you know enough about yourself and your constitution (*prakriti*)—your lifelong tendencies, characteristics and original traits—you will be able to pick what works best for you in order to come into balance. Ayurveda offers a system you can use to assess your constitution. This system is known as the *dosha* system. The doshas are the three elements that together, in different ratios, make up your prakriti*)*. The three doshas are *vata, pitta,* and *kapha.* We will look at each one in detail, once we test ourselves and know our own personal doshas (or our *prakriti*).

The flexitarian method offers many tools for achieving balance and bliss, and once you know your *prakriti*, it will be easier to decide which tools to choose and how to use them.

Test Yourself

Below you will find a questionnaire. Fill it out as accurately as possible, but don't get stuck on any particular questions. Just choose the answer that describes "in general" what you are most like, and then you can decide how strongly you want to identify with the statement. Of course, maybe the past week was unusual for you, but we are looking to identify the basic structure of our personality and body. There is no right or wrong answer. Some questions refer to your body, and those are pretty easy, while others refer to your personality. In those cases, just be as sincere as possible.

Prakriti: Know Your Body Type

Next to each question write a number from 1 to 5 that describes how much you agree with the statement. 1 = do not agree; 5 = totally agree. Try to answer in general and not necessarily only for recent times.

At the bottom, add up the total for each section. Remember there is no result that is better than another. Having more of one dosha (body element) compared with another is not better or worse, and having them all equally does not mean that you are balanced.

Section One—Vata

1. I tend to be thin and have sharp protruding bones.

2. I tend to have cold hands and feet.

3. I tend to have dry skin.

4. My hair tends to be on the dry side and can get frizzy easily.

5. My speech is quick and lively.

6. My movements are quick and sharp.

7. I am always on the go, ready for something new.

8. I learn new information rapidly.

9. I find it hard to remember all that I have to do.

10. I get excited easily.

11. I am spontaneous and open to trying new things.

12. I prefer warmer weather.

13. I get restless and agitated easily, needing to move or fidget.

14. I am full of ideas and tend to be creative.

15. My daily routine tends to vary, including meal and sleep times.

16. I tend to be sensitive and emotional.

17. I get stressed easily and tend to worry or get anxious.

18. I tend to have difficulty falling asleep.

19. I tend to eat quickly.

20. My digestion tends to be irregular with frequent gas or bloating.

Section Two—Pitta

1. I have a medium build and can get toned easily.

2. I have an intense gaze.

3. My hair is thin, shows early signs of graying, or is a reddish tone.

4. I am rational and a quick thinker.

5. I love making lists and crossing off completed tasks.

6. I am thorough in what I do.

7. I love taking on new projects.

8. I get very involved in what I do and can maintain focus on a task.

9. I aim for perfection and keep high standards.

10. I don't like to compromise and can be strong-willed.

11. I can get irritated and impatient easily.

12. I do things with passion and energy.

13. I get angry easily.

14. My friends say I am intense.

15. I sleep well and am fine with less than eight hours of sleep.

16. I heat up easily and prefer cooler environments.

17. I have a strong appetite and can eat large quantities if I desire.

18. I get irritated if I don't eat when I am hungry.

19. I have a tendency to get heartburn.

20. I can be critical and argumentative.

Section Three—Kapha

1. I have a wider build with bigger bones.

2. I gain weight easily and have a hard time losing it.

3. My hair is full and on the oily side.

4. My skin is smooth and soft.

5. I am a loyal friend and devoted in my relationships.

6. People tend to confide in me.

7. I am forgiving and sweet natured in general.

8. I am slow to move and move slowly.

9. I am not excited about doing physical activity.

10. I am a good listener, and speaking is not a natural trait.

11. I tend to hold emotions inside.

12. I tend to withdraw instead of confront.

13. I don't like to let go of things even if I don't expect to use them again.

14. I have difficulty leaving a relationship, even after it is no longer nourishing.

15. I don't like change, and enjoy a steady routine.

16. I have good endurance.

17. I do my tasks slowly and steadily.

18. I learn slowly but retain information well.

19. I like sleeping, and eight hours is not a lot, in my opinion.

20. I have a hard time getting up in the morning and starting my day.

Total Section One/Vata:

Total Section Two/Pitta:

Total Section Three/Kapha:

WHAT DOES THIS MEAN?

You now have three numbers next to the three words *vata, pitta,* and *kapha.* These are your doshas, the three elements of your prakriti. Understanding the doshas will be our road map to understanding our selves.

We all have some of each dosha within us. What makes us unique is the ratio of the three in our body. There is no ideal ratio. By no means is having all three doshas equal better in any way than having one dosha much more dominant, and another much lower. It is about having each dosha balanced within itself (or within us) that brings us into a place of harmony. It is common to find two more dominant doshas with one dosha a bit less prominent.

According to tradition, our doshas are pretty much constant. Your prakriti or original constitution is basically inherited. I am, and always was, pitta dominant with a strong vata and a lower kapha. Pitta-vata would be the way to express it. As I've grown older my kapha has gone up and my pitta does not come in as high. What really happened is that I managed to calm down some of the flare-ups I used to have. Part of the reason the score has changed is that I answered the questions according to myself at that specific time, and not according to who I was as a toddler. (Honestly, I don't remember myself in such detail back then; do you?) So my solution is to try to answer the questions according to my tendencies in general. Maybe today I am less angry than I used to be, but I can understand the intensity of anger, as it has always been part of me.

Ayurvedic doctors use pulse checking and other systems to get more accurate "readings" of our bodies. This questionnaire will be our main tool. Afterward, we will learn about each dosha separately—what is it like in and out of balance, as well as different ways to bring it back into balance. We can experience great change when the doshas come into balance. Many things can throw us out of balance: food, the climate, lifestyle, stress, pollution, and the way we think.

The Five Elements

There are five basic elements that make up this world: space, air, fire, water, and earth. In Ayurveda, we look at what the elements represent and how they function, rather than what they actually are. These elements are the same as those that make up our own bodies. The doshas, the psycho-physiological energies of our bodies, are mainly a combination of two of the elements. Thus the doshas within us exist in harmony within nature. These are the five elements used in Ayurveda:

Space: a field through which all other fields can manifest;

Air: a gaseous state of matter, an existence without form;

Fire: a power that can convert solid to liquid and gas, a form with no substance, always in a state of transformation;

Water: a liquid state of matter, a substance with no stability unless it is contained;

Earth: a solid state of matter; stability.

Each dosha has two elements: vata: space and air; pitta: fire and water; kapha: water and earth.

We Contain All of the Doshas and All Elements within Us

The doshas are variable and tend to shift according to our surroundings, nutritional status, state of mind, stress level, activity level, and many other factors. Thus, they can move out of balance. When a dosha becomes extreme, more pronounced, and overly dominant at a level that brings discomfort to oneself or one's surroundings, it has moved away from balance and is in disharmony. For most of us, the doshas are constantly shifting slightly in one direction and then back. It is not uncommon, though, to have the shift out of balance continue, creating more unwanted effects on our bodies and mind. For some, this shift can go to extremes and create chronic illnesses or more severe cases of disease. The good news is that we can come back into balance and, over time, learn how to remain in a state of balance and equanimity

Vata Dosha: Control of Movement

The vata dosha is represented by air and space. It is the moving dosha. The vata dosha is responsible for our circulatory system, the impulses that trigger our nervous system, and the movement of our mind. In some ways, vata is considered to be the most influential of the three doshas because it is the moving force behind the other two doshas, which are incapable of movement without it. Vata dosha is responsible for all somatic activities and sensations. Vata is a powerful mediator between the outer world, and our perception and interpretation of that world. Vata channels everything we perceive (sound, smell, taste, sight, touch) through the appropriate sensory organs and, via the mind, processes and interprets them into the appropriate response of an organ or an action.

Vata is the air dosha, and thus breath and lungs are dominated by it, as well as the flow of nutrients, flatulence, gout, rheumatism, etc. We can very easily notice when vata is out of balance, as it has a great influence on our overall physical functioning through regulating the nervous processes of the body, mind, and emotional activity.

Characteristics of Vata Dominant Body Types

The vata dosha person is easily spotted physically as she will tend to be thin, with a slender body, bony, very tall or short, with relatively thin hair. The skin and hair will be on the dry side. Vata people need to use more creams and moisturizers. They may have long thin fingers and, in general, the classic ballerina look. Since they tend to be thin, they also suffer from cold hands and feet, and tend to seek warmer temperatures. Within a group of people, the vata person will normally be bundled up more than the others, or show signs of being cold. Vata personalities tend to walk more quickly, with short steps. They are the ones hurrying out the house, and forgetting where they put their keys. They are not the most orderly people, and find many things to be "cool."

Their appetite is irregular, and they may suffer from bloating or other digestive issues. They are light sleepers and may suffer from insomnia.

Vata personality is very creative, rich with new ideas, spontaneous, and free spirited— the artist type. They like change and get bored easily. They talk fast, think fast, and at times talk in a higher pitch, as they are easily excited and enthusiastic about their ideas.

The love of change also includes the love of movement—from movement with their bodies, to traveling, and changing lifestyles—they are always on the go. Vata personalities tend to be generous, joyful, full of vitality, open and outgoing. They love people, socializing, and going out—unbound.

Causes for Imbalanced Vata

There are certain situations and things that can cause the vata dominant personality to get out of balance. Though the vata person likes change and movement, in excess, this can cause them to go out of balance. Long commutes to work, frequent air travel, changes in lifestyle, such as change of work place, change of residency, and changes in relationships and friendships; even frequent changes in daily routine can be bad for the vata person.

Cold weather and dry wind also affect the vata person. If they do not have warm showers or baths, and moisturizers to balance this, they will go out of balance.

Any situation that is overly stimulating may be of excitement to the vata person, but since they are easily excited, they tend to go out of balance in such situations. Loud noise, big shopping malls, crowded places, flickering lights such as in casinos, abundant advertisements, and simply crowded streets like in NYC, can throw the vata person out of balance. This also includes excess mental stimulation.

Irregular diet, including fasting, eating lots of leftovers, eating at varied times, eating dry food, cold or frozen food, drinking ice cold drinks, as well as caffeine, smoking, drugs, sugar and alcohol are not good for the vata personality.

Emotionally challenging situations affect the vata person more than others. Fear, grief, depression, and anxiety-promoting situations will affect the vata person quickly.

If they do not get enough sleep, rest, and quiet time, if they are constantly in stimulating environments, the vata person will suffer. The opposite, such as too much exercise, or unbalanced workouts, with fast movements, that have no rest afterward will also throw the vata person out of balance.

Perhaps the worst in today's environment is the Internet. A vata person can easily skip between too many open windows on their computer, and easily get distracted with all the stimulations, pop-up windows, and offerings that the Internet can offer.

Signs That Your Vata Is out of Balance

In order to keep your vata balanced, you first need to know that it is out of balance. The vata person can be out of balance, and easily not know it. Many times they get addicted to the imbalanced life and do not recognize what is the cause of the unbalance. In the body, the vata person is overly dry—dry hair with split ends, dry skin, constant scratching, dry, chapped lips, and even a dry throat and dry cough can be present. Their digestion and elimination are irregular and disturbed; they may experience bloating, constipation, or gas. Less than one bowel movement each day may be a sign of vata imbalance. If the vata person is having a hard time focusing and paying attention, concentrating, or sitting still, is constantly fidgeting, moving, and feeling on the edge, there is an imbalance. They may be confused, agitated, forgetful, or spaced out. When they are feeling worried, anxious, overwhelmed, or emotionally challenged, they tend to be out of balance.

When the vata person is over excited, their voice tends to have a higher pitch and become much faster, and their breath shallow and quick. Though they love change, when vata people are constantly on the go, even when they are tired, and feel like they just can't stop, or even slow down, no matter how tired they are—this is a sign they have gone too far. On the other hand, when they feel lethargic, with very low energy, and no enthusiasm for life, this is the other side of an imbalanced vata. Maybe this leads to insomnia, light or interrupted sleep—all signs that vata is out of balance. These are all symptoms of the mind out of balance, which is the classic vata imbalance. This includes being forgetful, and a feeling of lost control over life.

You could be mostly pitta or kapha and still have a vata imbalance. If you find that you are showing more pronounced signs of vata than usual, then you need to balance your vata. Vata dosha is the first dosha to come out of balance, as it is the moving dosha. If you can identify with many of the statements above, following a vata-balancing diet and lifestyle can help bring vata back to balance.

BALANCING VATA WITH FOOD AND NUTRITION

Food and nutrition affect us tremendously, and since the vata personality tends to eat whatever is around, without too much care about when and what, it is especially important to take care and eat right for balancing the vata dosha.

Vata does well with warm grounding foods, such as root vegetables, soups (carrot soup, pureed butternut soup, etc.), stews, and casseroles. Warm grains such as quinoa, brown rice, spelt, and millet may be included, as well. Vegetables or tempeh (fermented soy cutlets), cooked in warm water or sauce are good. In general, cooking with moisture is good for vata. Sweet potatoes, parsnips, green beans, winter squash, asparagus, and other dense vegetables are good for grounding vata.

Decrease consumption of vegetables from the nightshade family, such as eggplant, potatoes, tomatoes, and peppers. You can eat them in moderation if needed, and better if they are cooked. Avoid large beans. Beans are cold, dry, and heavy—not the attributes that support vata. Use fresh ginger root, cilantro, parsley, fresh basil, fresh fennel, mint, rosemary, thyme, and oregano for spicing up your food. For dry spices, use warming spices (cinnamon, nutmeg, cayenne, turmeric, mustard seeds, coriander, cumin, cloves, black pepper, lemon and orange zest, rock salt, or sea salt), and such oils as sesame, olive oil, and ghee (clarified butter).

Though nuts may be grounding, they are also dry and can irritate vata. Eat nuts preferably soaked and unsalted, such as almonds. Also fine are cashews, walnuts, pistachios, hazelnuts, pecans, pine nuts, sesame seeds, sunflower seeds, and pumpkin seeds.

Eat vata-balancing fruits: avocados, pineapples, papayas, peaches, plums, grapes, mangoes, oranges, cherries, berries, limes, lemons, coconut, fresh figs, and raisins (soaked).

Consume warm drinks with no caffeine, such as rice or nut milks, herbal tea, warm water, and lemon-ginger-honey tea. Avoid dry foods such as crackers and dry cereal. They may aggravate vata. To balance this, drink plenty of warm drinks between meals. To balance your vata, eat warm, grounding food and reduce sugars, including bread and alcohol. Eat calmly and in non-stimulating surroundings. Chew slowly and focus on your food.

Balancing Vata with Lifestyle

Having a consistent daily routine is one of the first steps to balancing vata. Try to rise and go to bed at the same time, and follow a reasonable, steady schedule, including consistent meal times. You may start your day the same every day, with setting an intention and meditation. This will help keep your mind clear and clean for the day.

Eat slowly, chew well, and dine in relaxing settings. Vatas tend to hurry up and just swallow. Do not eat in front of your computer, and if possible, try not to have conversations while eating. In short—just eat. Take a moment after your meal to sit and breathe. Slowing down and allowing your food to begin its digestion process in the mouth will help improve digestion throughout the body.

Take an oil massage before you shower. This will help with circulation, keeping the skin moisturized and nourished, and will help relax the muscles and nerves. Use almond, sesame, or jojoba oil. Warm up some oil briefly in a pan. Massage the oil onto your skin in long movements over the limbs, and in circular movements toward the center of the body and over the joints. Let the oil sit on your body for ten to twenty minutes. (Brush your teeth, do gentle head and shoulder rotations, or just sit and meditate on a towel while you wait.) Then take a shower using very mild soap. (I like Dr. Bronner's soap as it already contains oils.) Ideally do this every day, but realistically maybe three to four times a week. I find that unless I need to bring more balance into my life, doing it even once a week has a great effect. In the winter, it is best to do it a bit more often, as the skin tends to dry out more. On days when you have not done the oil massage, use a moisturizer after showering. Unrefined organic sesame oil works great. Use lip balm to keep the lips moist.

Vata has a tendency to get cold, and yet still not dress appropriately. Stay warm; in the winter it is especially important to wear layers, thick socks, and gloves when needed.

For exercise, take a twenty-minute walk, and then practice yoga in a slow, controlled manner.

Sleep is especially important for vata people. They have a tendency to be excited about life, a conversation that is happening, or to simply be running within their own minds. Sleep well. Try to get to bed early, before 10:00 pm or as early as you need to, in order to get rest and restore the movement of vata.

Perhaps one of the most important lifestyle practices for vata, and probably one of the most challenging, is meditation. Learning to slow down, to allow the mind to quiet, and to be able to see the mind as an observer, allows the vata person to take control of the emotionally challenging situations in life. It is especially important to set a timer and decide to stay put for twenty minutes, as the vata mind will find excuses galore why it is time to stop (or not begin in the first place).

Remember, slow down, move less, and find activities that help you focus and relax. Keep warm and cozy, and avoid places of distractions. Do one thing at a time!

Balancing Vata with Yoga Asana

Movement is very pleasant for the vata person, and is a good way to come to balance, if done correctly. Have a slow, steady, calm and consistent practice, preferably at the same time each day, as a routine. Focus on grounding and strengthening, getting into poses slowly, and holding steady for longer periods of time. Use even inhales and exhales, or allow the exhales to be deeper. This will help the mind slow down, and the body to stay calm. Begin with slow sun salutes, emphasizing deep, full breaths and conscious movement, and then practice slow standing poses held for longer periods of time, focusing on grounding. Practice standing balancing poses, especially tree, to cultivate steadiness. Try to hold for ten breaths each side.

On the floor, practice spinal stretching and bending in all directions, especially forward folds, and hip openers, such as pigeon and baddha konasana. When practicing backbends, go slowly (I think by now you understand the main point is to slow down and breath deeply and calmly), and make sure to take a short rest after poses, and then maybe add twists, forward folds, or child's pose. When practicing inversions, try to hold them steadily and for longer periods. Use the wall if necessary. And maybe the most important pose for vata people is savasana. Skipping savasana is one of the most vata-unbalancing options. Consider staying in savasana for ten to fifteen minutes.

Whatever you do, do it slowly. Breathe deeply and stay longer in the poses. Practice in non-distracting environments, preferably calm and quiet.

Vata is fun and happy, creative and spontaneous, your favorite friend to go out with, to share ideas with, and hear stories from. Vata people just need to make sure they slow down, breathe, and pay attention. It is too easy for them to get addicted to their unbalanced state and find excuses why it is okay to stay there. Practice awareness!

Pitta Dosha: Control of Metabolism

Pitta is fire and water, the fire of the digestive system, as well as the fire to digest our thoughts. It is what stimulates us to go, do, and move. It is the "type A" within us, the one that creates lists, that likes things to be well organized and under control, the go-getter. Pitta stimulates our ambition, enthusiasm, and determination. It is the furnace of the body, and the fire that breaks down our food into usable nutrients.

Characteristics of Pitta Dominant Body Types

The pitta person has a medium build with an athletic and toned body. They have penetrating eyes with excellent vision, a strong voice that can be heard from afar, and are articulate, argumentative, and persuasive. The hair is lustrous and usually slightly wavy, with a tendency to early graying and baldness. Their skin is soft, with a good complexion, healthy facial tone, and warm coloration, and if the skin is light, it tends to burn in the sun.

They have a strong appetite, good digestion, and fast metabolism, but lose patience when hungry. They have a purposeful stride, and high energy for short durations, which makes them good sprinters.

The pitta person tends to be determined, ambitious, precise, strong willed, courageous, and confident—an overachiever or type A personality. They like having tasks and projects, and even more so, they like to complete the project. Lists are their best friends, and they take great pleasure in organizing them and checking off items that have been completed.

They tend to have a focused, sharp mind; they are alert and observant of details. They can concentrate when needed, are enthusiastic for knowledge, and love the use of logic. Their good memory helps them learn quickly in the subjects of their interest.

They are disciplined and responsible in life, and go about their tasks and activities with passion, but mostly at the beginning. They can be irritable, jealous, judgmental, and easy to anger, but also have a good sense of humor and are, in general, happy. They are initiators, but like to have things done their own way. They spend moderately, mostly on luxuries. Think of the entrepreneur, a self-confident, ambitious person with a medium build and a toned body.

Causes for Imbalanced Pitta

Since pitta has a lot of fire to begin with excess heat, hot climates, and hot times of day will cause them imbalances. Humidity, especially with heat, will also aggravate them. Since the pitta person tends to be a perfectionist, any form of criticism, being under pressure, excess work, and over thinking will cause excess pitta. They will also be out of balance when they are fatigued and lacking adequate sleep and rest. Negative emotions, fear, hate, and anger are major imbalance causes for the pitta person.

Too many hot foods, including spicy foods, too many cooked meals, a lack of fresh ingredients, excess caffeine, salt, sour food, oily food, fermented foods, red meat, and alcohol can all aggravate pitta. Nightshade will also aggravate pitta. The pitta person does not do well when hungry. They will need at least something small to calm the burning digestive fire, or they may be very irritable. Drugs and especially antibiotics, as well as exercising at midday or in very hot environments, such as hot yoga, are not good for the pitta person.

Pitta is easily out of balance when over heated, whether from climate, food, or emotions.

Signs That Your Pitta Is out of Balance

Physically the pitta person will lose hair, when combing or even shampooing. They will suffer from heartburn or excess stomach acid. Inflammation, rashes, and ulcers are all signs of pitta imbalance. They will feel hotter than usual, be constantly thirsty, and may have red eyes.

An out of balance pitta person will feel impatient and irritable. Every little thing will be a trigger for them to get upset or angry. They will have low tolerance of other people, and feel provoked and frustrated. Their speech can turn intense or be sharp and sarcastic, at times even hurtful to others. They will become overly argumentative. (Who, me? Of course not.)

They may even experience uncontrollable anger, temper bursts, or times of intense speaking. Their passion for their projects will go overboard. They may be overworking, or obsessed with their project. At times they will keep going, forgoing sleep, forgetting to drink, skipping meals just to complete something. This sometimes leads them to wake up in the very early hours of the morning, and then having a hard time getting back to sleep. Be aware of your body temperature. If you feel hot in the body, spicy in your mouth, or heated emotionally, you have gone out of balance.

BALANCING PITTA WITH FOOD AND NUTRITION

Food is a good way to balance pitta. Eat foods that help you cool down, like raw foods. Eat some dry foods to balance the watery nature of pitta, and use healthy fats such as ghee, olive oil, and coconut oil. Eat sweet foods, such as brown rice, carrots, beets, sweet potatoes, parsnips, squash, and fruit such as pears, pineapple, and mangoes (including small amounts of dried fruit), but avoid all refined sugars. Eat bitter and astringent foods such as greens, broccoli, cauliflower, green beans, asparagus, artichoke, mung beans, and Brussels sprouts. Eat these with some grains, such as quinoa, oats, rice, barley, and amaranth.

Eat fewer salty, pungent, and sour foods (which is what you will crave). Cereal, crackers, soaked almonds, sunflower seeds, pumpkin seeds, and healthy energy bars (especially with almonds and dates) can be good snack choices. Avoid overly hot spices. Turmeric, cumin, cinnamon, cardamom, and fennel are good choices as well as cooling herbs such as mint, basil, and thyme.

Eat fruit and cereal for breakfast (cooked fruit can work well in the winter); green smoothies are fantastic always. Make your lunch the main meal, and eat a light dinner.

Drink small amounts of fruit juice diluted with water, sparkling water, or small amounts of coconut water (it is very sweet, so it's best to sip it over longer periods of time). Drink smoothies made with fruits, almonds, coconut, and dates. Add some kale or bok-choi to balance the sweet and get the health benefits of dark leafy greens. Drink sufficient amounts of water between meals; the water should be room temperature or slightly cool, but not ice cold.

BALANCING PITTA WITH LIFESTYLE

Stay cool, especially emotionally; don't let things get to you. Walk away from situations that will cause you to get fired up. Avoid going out in the heat of the day, especially on an empty stomach or after you have eaten tangy or spicy foods. Stay cool physically; avoid exercising when it's hot. Find activities that are not competitive. Spend time around water. Go swimming; walk near water, streams, rivers, or the beach when the weather is not too hot. Go to sleep early, no later than 10:30 pm if possible. Drink a small amount of warm almond milk with cardamom and a bit of honey before bedtime.

Stay balanced. Make time for rest and rejuvenation on a daily basis. Know when to stop working. When you do take breaks, make sure you are away from your cell phone and computer. Do not wait too long to take a break, as the tendency is to think you are still doing well, until it is too late.

All relaxation activities are good for balancing pitta. Take Ayurvedic oil with coconut oil, and most importantly, meditate! It will help you stay cool emotionally and keep you balanced. Two words for pitta people: stay cool! Both in and out. Don't take things personally, and don't get upset about things that don't matter too much.

Balancing Pitta with Yoga Asana

Practice in a non-competitive, nurturing environment. Do not practice in a heated room over 85 degrees Fahrenheit. Practice long exhalations to relax, calm, and cool the body. Bring awareness to your body to release tension in the muscles after challenging poses. Soften your gaze (drsti), and relax the intensity in your face when doing strong or challenging poses. Enjoy standing poses that open the hips, and practice seated twists and forward folds, especially those that open the hips. Backbends can increase pitta, as they tend to be intense. Try to practice them just to the point where you can still breathe deeply and stay calm. Make sure to follow with cooling twists and forward folds. Headstand is a warming pose, so if practicing headstand, be steady and breathe deeply to maintain coolness. Shoulder stand is a cooling alternative. Finish your practice with cooling poses and calming pranayama. In pranayama, breathe deeply, emphasizing left nostril breathing as this activates the right side of the brain, as well as the relaxation response in the body. When needed, practice cooling breathing techniques to lower body temperature, but also to calm emotions, asthma, or acidic stomach.

Really make sure your environment is supportive for you to stay cool. Resist the temptation to practice too hard and too intensely, and be okay with wherever you are.

The pitta is your favorite friend to organize an event or party. They will take a project and make it happen. Let them plan your travels, your wedding, or go over your business plan. But remember, pitta needs to stop, rest, and calm down. Keep it cool!

Kapha Dosha: Control of Structure

Kapha is water and earth, grounded and stable, lubricated, fluid yet heavy, moving slowly. The kapha person is the calm, slow-moving, larger body frame, and pretty chill person that you would like to have as your friend. They are steady, cool, and happy to stay for another drink, once you actually get them out of their home. Kapha is like a rock—steady, strong, reliable, happy to stay still, and always there when you need them.

Characteristics of Kapha Dominant Body Types

Kapha bodies tend to have a broad frame with thick, long limbs, with a good, strong, solid, supportive neck. They are strong, with firm musculature, thick bones, and good stamina and endurance. Marathon runners tend to have some kapha in them. They tend to gain weight easily and have a hard time losing the extra pounds. Their appetite is constant but poor.

They have rich, silky, dense, and smooth hair. Their skin is thick, oily, pale, and cold, and they tend to have large, full, rounded face and lips, with healthy teeth and gums.

Their stride may be slow, but it is a steady one. On the dance floor, they may not seem like wild dancers, but they can stay for a very long time. Same goes with their sex drive—strong and enduring. They are great listeners, and do not say much. When they do speak, they speak slowly and evenly, with a low voice.

Kapha people love sleeping. They sleep deeply and for long periods of time, and have a hard time getting out of bed.

They are mostly pleasant, calm, faithful, reliable, stable, loyal, easy-going, supportive, and patient people with deep and resonant voices. They are grounded, centered, stable, supportive, caring, and compassionate. They do not anger easily, but once they do, it's hard for them to calm down.

The kapha person may be lethargic and even lazy. They may learn slowly, but they have good memories. They take time before reaching a conclusion and are great with logical analysis. The kapha person is your best friend. Steady, reliable, and consistent. I think of the voluptuous woman, with beautiful, rich, wavy hair, that gives you a perfect smile, who makes you feel at home at once.

Causes for Imbalanced Kapha

Since the kapha person does not like change or movement, a sedentary lifestyle is the worst for them. Other ways a kapha person can go out of balance are: not enough exercise and movement; doing nothing; gazing at the TV; using sedatives or tranquilizers; not enough mental stimulation and challenge; not enough variety in life; repetitive actions, slowness, and inertia.

Too many fats and oily foods in the diet, including cooking oil, fried and deep fried foods, dairy products, and meat will cause increased heaviness and lethargy. So will too much bread and sweets, iced foods and iced drinks, or even excessive amounts of drinking water. Exposure to cold weather, napping after meals, and over-sleeping will imbalance the kapha person.

Doubts, greed, lack of companionship, and possessiveness or hoarding will take the kapha out of balance. Stagnation, no movement, lack of stimulation, both physical and mental, are the root causes for an imbalanced kapha; the couch potato.

Signs That Your Kapha Is out of Balance

Your kapha is out of balance when you gain weight easily, even without having much of an appetite; feeling tired and lethargic for no apparent reason; having a hard time waking up, even after sufficient hours of sleep. You may also feel tired when you wake up, not wanting to get out of bed. During the day, the couch appears very appealing and it's hard to get off of it. You may have trouble getting motivated and be resistant to change even when you know it is the right thing for you—you would rather keep things as they are, feeling attached, clingy, jealous or insecure, mentally unmotivated, not very talkative—you would rather watch and be an observer.

When feeling ill, you may notice a heavy and congested throat, head, or chest. Skin is breaking out or is very oily, and hair is oily, even after shampooing. Your digestion is slow, and you feel heavy and lethargic after meals. The best word to describe the feeling of a kapha out of balance is heaviness. When the zest for life is gone, kapha went overboard.

BALANCING KAPHA WITH FOOD AND NUTRITION

Eat meals regularly. You do not need large quantities, but make sure you do not skip a meal. Eat less oily food, less fat, less salt, and less sweet. Instead, add more fresh herbs and pungent, astringent, and bitter foods such as carrots, asparagus, okra, bitter leafy greens, and cruciferous vegetables (broccoli, cauliflower, Brussels sprouts, daikon, kale). Steam them lightly to help with digestion. Avoid nightshades (potatoes, eggplants, tomatoes, peppers).

Eat grains in moderation, and choose lighter whole grains. Barley, buckwheat, millet, and quinoa are good choices. If you choose heavier grains, such as rice or wheat, eat very small quantities. Eat yogurt and fermented foods such as sauerkraut; they will help with your digestion. Sprouts are also a good choice, and if you like beans, eat small ones such as mung beans, preferably sprouted.

Use turmeric, cumin, coriander, cayenne, black pepper, ginger, cloves, and fenugreek for their flavor, aroma, and healing properties. Eat fewer snacks, but if needed, rice cakes, crackers with low salt, and cereal are good choices Use honey when a sweetener is needed, or simply eat fresh fruit such as apples, melons, and berries, preferably between meals.

Drink a lot of warm water. You can add ginger, lemon, and a bit of honey. Think light; think raw, think of sprouts. Enjoy all the foods that are bursting with energy, fresh and alive. Skip the fats and sugars.

Balancing Kapha with Lifestyle

Exercise every day and include some exercise that is vigorous. Get up and move around every few hours, preferably in the fresh air.

Try some challenging mental activity; for example, get a Sudoku book, or learn a new language. Travel to new places, even if it scares you. Explore new activities, go to museums or galleries, try new restaurants, and find new routes to work. Meet new people, engage in conversations, and volunteer to be active.

Do skin scrubs and exfoliate to get rid of impurities. Make sure you go to sleep early, and get up very early, before the sun. Do not take naps; instead, meditate for thirty minutes daily.

To sum it up in one word—move! Any way you like it, just move; move your body and stimulate your mind.

Balancing Kapha with Yoga Asana

Have an active and warming practice to stimulate metabolism and circulation. Take deep breaths with emphasis on inhalation to keep your fire alive. Practice challenging poses that produce heat and sweat, such as backbends—especially bow pose (*dhanurasana*), as it stimulates pitta. Add to the mix core-work arm balances and inversions, such as forearm balance (*pincha mayurasana*) and handstand. Try a strong flowing practice that goes a bit beyond your instinct to take a break.

Practice extra sun salutes to increase your heart rate, take an extra chaturanga to kindle your fire, and spend less time in downward dog. Practice warrior poses, especially warrior 1, and take variations that open the chest. Do the standing twists, and then add some seated twists as well. Practice a fierce pose (*utkatasana*) with intense pranayama (power breath), such as *kapalabhati* (breath of fire). Practice seated poses for shorter periods of time to avoid cooling and creating lethargy. Consider taking a vinyasa between each pose, and add a few rounds of heating breath work (*pranayama*) such as *kapalabhati* and *bhastrika*. Any yoga that will be challenging, gets you moving and your heart rate up, makes you sweat and challenges your breath, will be good for you.

The kapha is lucky to have a steady, calm personality in today's fast-moving world. However, kapha should really watch out for the tendency to become a couch potato. With steady practices of movement such as yoga, running, biking, dancing, swimming, and the like, the kapha person can guarantee she will stay active, fit, and avoid the tendency to gain weight and be lethargic. Chose some non-kapha friends to stimulate excitement and movement.

PART 2

The Four Elements
of the Method

Now that you know more about yourself, where you may have a tendency to go out of balance, and some basic lifestyle practices to get you going—it is time to dive into the heart of the flexitarian method, which is the foundation of a healthy and happy yoga lifestyle.

Part 2 presents you with the four elements of the flexitarian method. We will start with the yoga asana (yoga poses), where you will learn more about your body, about the poses and their groupings, as well as some sample yoga sequences to begin working with.

Then we will move into the pranayama (breath work) chapter, where you will learn a variety of practices to increase the energy in the body, balance your emotions and brain, create heat or cool down, and really support the yoga asanas. These two chapters go hand in hand.

Next we will learn about food and nutrition, which are the foundation for a healthy life and help support a healthy body to do yoga and pranayama, as well as the mind, since what we eat affects our mental state as well.

We will finish the section with the fourth element—mediation and mind training. When the mind is in balance and peace, all other layers of life—including the first three elements of the flexitarian method—flow better and achieve better results.

This is your practical practice chapter, where we start to live the yoga lifestyle. Practice with patience, reduce expectations, and the results will show. Just keep showing up, and be your authentic self.

— 4 —

Physical Yoga

Yoga is the state of no activity in the mind, a state of bliss, where there is no more suffering, and our daily circumstances do not affect us anymore. Sometimes it is referred to as a state of liberation, of freedom from our thinking mind.

Since this is not an easy state to achieve simply by our own will, many practices were developed to help us achieve this state. In this section we will look at the practices of *hatha yoga*—physical practices that use our body and breath to get healthier and more focused—to help us gain better control of our body and mind, and eventually enter a state of bliss. The yogis of the past were concerned with all layers of the being, including food and diet. They ate healthy food that kept their bodies healthy and balanced; this in turn helped them keep a healthy mind. It is much harder to work on the mind when we have a backache or a cold. So the yoga practices are aimed at maintaining vitality and health, so we can further work on our minds with ease.

There are many debates as to how old yoga is or when it began, but it is known for sure that yoga in one form or another was practiced many centuries ago. Traditional yoga answers questions such as "Who am I? Where do I come from? Where do I go? What must I do?" in a way similar to many religions and philosophical practices.

The masters of ceremony in the old days had to practice focus and concentration while performing their duties and, at times, they had visions that transcended the ordinary mind. These masters were called *rishis*—the seers—and their practices are the roots of yogic practices today.

What Are the Benefits of Yoga?

Yoga is a practice intended to lead us to a more blissful life, with a healthy body and a calm and focused mind. The practice of yoga helps us understand who we really are, and how to transverse the perceptions of the mind.

Some Benefits of Yoga in Brief

Benefits many body systems. Improves digestion with twists and pranayama. Cleanses the body of waste by stimulating the lymphatic system. Improves circulation. Improves lung efficiency with pranayama practice, which allows us to use our lungs more efficiently. Cleanses through breath work such as *kapalabhati.* Strengthens the immune system by stimulating the parasympathetic nervous system.

Improves flexibility and strength. Keeps the spine supple, especially when bending backward and twisting. Relieves back pains and stiffness by stretching the back in all six directions. Improves posture by stretching and lengthening the spine, and opening the chest and shoulders. Improves flexibility by increasing range of motion throughout every single joint. Improves stamina and energy. Tones muscles by extending them as they work, resulting in a lean—rather than buff—look. Invites courage and empowers us when we manifest a new pose or learn to do an inversion or arm balance. Balancing practices create balance through better body awareness, from standing on one leg to holding a crescent pose steadily.

Has a balancing and calming effect. Relaxes the body and calms the mind, especially by the deepening of the breath. Improves sleep, not only thanks to the physical activity, but also the breath work and calming of the mind. Relieves stress, even if temporarily, with breath work and chanting. Balances energy channels throughout the body with pranayama practices; cultivates balance between the left and right sides of the brain.

The benefits of yoga can be felt in the body, the breath, and the mind. One of the greatest benefits is attaining a sense of bliss beyond your conscious mind. Keep practicing with no attachment to the results, and the fruit will appear on its own.

In this section, you will learn some physical practices that will help you become stronger, more flexible, and leaner; you will learn how to tone your muscles and develop your lungs. The practices will also help with your digestion and overall health, as these poses activate different hormones in the body (including the feel-good ones), and promote healthy circulation of blood, lymphatic fluid, and energy in the body.

The practice of yoga poses (specifically my method called Doron Yoga, which I'll share with you here) is based on the foundation of traditional yoga—mostly ashtanga vinyasa as taught by Pattabhi Jois—but blends in contemporary knowledge of anatomy, alignment, and other modalities that can help promote an overall sense of physical well-being. It balances yin with yang—at times moving vigorously to get stronger, and at times holding poses longer to gain calm and flexibility. The Doron Yoga method is a balanced vinyasa system where movements flow from one to another in rhythm with the breath, emphasizing grace as the way to open to a meditative practice. The practice is practical, non-dogmatic, and sustainable; it protects the body from injuries and creates a place where the mind can surrender and soften while the body can strengthen and energize. The practice works with breath, flexibility, strength, and focus. Doron Yoga is a complete and efficient method for cultivating awareness, compassion, strength, and sensitivity, leading to a transformation to inner freedom. This blends smoothly with the other three elements of the flexitarian method. The breathing practices help the ease of movement, and the openness of the body prepares for the breathing practices. Some are incorporated with the yoga poses. This practice is a form of mind training, and helps with the deeper, more still, meditation practices.

The Practice of Doron Yoga

- Move with ease. Balance your effort with calmness.
- Breath as you move. Inhale as you open, lift up, or rise to standing, and exhale as you lower down or forward fold.
- Keep awareness alive as you move. Follow the movements of your body with your gaze so you remain focused. Listen to the sound of your breath, and stay attentive to what is happening in your body.

- Have fun! Yes, it may be hard at times, but remind yourself of your goal, so you can stay focused, and then surrender to the pleasure of the process.

Tristana—the Three Essentials

Tristana is the foundation—the supporting pillars—of the practice of ashtanga and vinyasa yoga, and as such, it is the tool to help cultivate the ultimate presence of mind, focus, and stability of the body and mind. The tools are breath *(ujjayi)*, gaze *(drsti)* and control centers *(bandhas)*. These tools work synergistically to enhance our experience as we practice. The breath and the gaze keep us focused and present. The gaze and the control centers help us stay balanced as well as deepen our postures; the control centers and the breath help maintain the energy level of the body. It is with these tools that we transform our asana practice from a simple body exercise into a complete mind-body transformation, from a huffing and puffing workout into a graceful flow. Tristana connects our physical yoga with our energetic breathing and our mind training. Now just eat well before you practice, and you have integrated all of the flexitarian practices into your day.

Ujjayi Breath—Ocean Breath (Victorious Breath)

One of the most important aspects of yoga is breathing. The fundamental technique of yogic breathing is ujjayi breath, or "victorious" breath. It is the foundation for many other pranayama techniques, works in synergy with yogic gaze (*drsti*) to help focus the mind, and the yoga control centers, or power centers (*bandhas*), to keep the energetic flow (prana) in the body. It is also an important practice on its own.

Ujjayi breathing has many benefits. It slows down and lengthens the breath. By filling up the lungs entirely, ujjayi increases lung capacity, and helps increase the supply of breath and oxygen in the muscles to help with the movements we do in yoga. It is a point of concentration or focus for the mind that aids us in the practice of *pratyahara* (withdrawal of the senses) and keeps the mind steady and calm, especially when poses get challenging.

Ujjayi practice is done by drawing the breath in and out through the nose, while slightly constricting the opening of the throat where air passes through the glottis. Though the air does enter and exit through the nose, most of the awareness and sensation is at the throat. That is why sometimes ujjayi is known as throat breathing, or ocean breath. It is the friction of air through the glottis that produces an ocean wave-like sound. This sound is known as *ajapa mantra*, the unspoken mantra.

Practice ujjayi breath first in a comfortable seated position. Try to equalize the inhalations and exhalations. Once you have mastered ujjayi breath while seated, you can start to use it in your asana practice by synchronizing your movement with the breath. During the transitions of *asana* practice, work on regulating the breath to match the movement, keeping the breath flowing calmly and with ease. Strenuous breathing may mean that you need to back off, either with the physical body or with the attitude of the mind.

Off your yoga mat, ujjayi breath can be practiced anywhere at any time. It is an excellent way to relax, calm the mind, focus, and alleviate insomnia.

Bandhas—Energy Locks or Control Centers

Bandha means to bind or to lock. We are physically and energetically activating parts of our body that help maintain and regulate all internal systems, as well as our internal energy. These locks are located at energy centers in our body. As we learn to use them, we learn deeper control and stability, improve focus and centeredness, regulate deeper breaths, and maintain a calmer mind. You can think of bandhas as control centers—as activation and regulation centers—so as we create these locks, we are controlling the energy and body systems, which help maintain control of body and mind.

The *bandhas* are key in asana practice. Beyond the energy in the body, which of course helps the energy of the pose, the *bandhas* also help create support for the spine and lower back during transitions, creating the "lightness" and graceful appearance of some of the more challenging poses, such as arm balances or the jump-through.

The two *bandhas* we will use are *mulabandha* (root control center) and *uddiyanabandha* (flying up control center).

Mulabandha (Root Energy Lock, Root Control Center)

The root bandha sits at the root of the spine. Lifting the pelvic floor helps activate it. At first you may lift more than what is needed, including the tightening of the anus, but as you refine your practice, you will learn to activate just the necessary muscles.

Try to slow down the flow of urine while using the toilet without using your abs, gluteus or leg muscles; you are probably using the correct muscles. If you are a woman, imagine that you are out and about, when you feel that your period has arrived a day early. The muscles you use to hold it in are the same muscles you use to activate mulabandha. For men, imagine it as lifting a diamond-shaped hammock between the anus and genitals and stretching it as well between the two sitting bones. Mulabandha is not easy to find and keep, but when we learn to activate it, it is powerful far beyond its physicality, as it is located at the root of the energy source. Mulabandha helps with the stability of the poses and serves as a strong foundation for all movement in the body. It evokes uddiyanabandha (see below) to action and stimulates energy to rise.

Uddiyanabandha (Flying Up Energy Lock)

Uddiyanabandha sits about two fingers' width below the navel. It is activated by lifting the belly in and up. The lifting is done in a gentle way; you should still be able to breathe fully. The traverse abdominal muscles (inner abdominal muscles) will be activated. Uddiyanabandha is engaged during asana practice to help support the lower back and strengthen the core. It also helps lengthen the lower back, so that there is more space between the vertebrae, especially L4 and L5. This in turn helps support the whole torso so it can stay steady, thus protecting the lower back. This is important in all poses, but it is especially noticed in standing balancing poses, as well as arm balances and inversions. Uddiyanabandha maintains the energy rising up toward the heart energy center.

Drsti—Point of Focus

The practice of drsti, or yogic gaze, is used to help us practice both focus and stability; it leads us to the concentration needed to keep us balanced and helps control the tendency to wander around following our senses. Drsti is a perfect aid in the practice of *pratyahara* (withdrawal of the senses), and it initiates the practice of *dharana* (concentration).

There are nine drsti points, and each pose has its own prescribed drsti. Some of the drsti points not only help with focus, but actually help us go deeper into the pose, such as in twists, when we take our gaze far to the side we are twisting toward. Other times the gaze helps us stay grounded, or in the case of supine twists, when taking the gaze in the direction opposite of the legs, drsti helps to ground the opposite shoulder and thus aids in getting a fuller twist in the entire back. It is not as crucial that you keep your gaze at a specific prescribed point as it is to keep your gaze very steady and aware—aware of what you are looking at.

Tristana is the secret to a graceful yoga practice. When all three elements of tristana are working together, the yoga practice flows with greater ease, focus, stability, and concentration. When you see videos of yogis flowing through powerful practices with apparent ease, it is the power of ujjayi, drsti, and bandhas that make the difference.

Yoga *Asana* Practice

The benefits of yoga asana practice are many, on the physical plane, as well as on the mind and spiritual planes. The clearest benefit is physical—you will notice greater flexibility and balance, improved joint mobility, stronger and leaner muscles, and you will lose fat, increase stamina, improve posture and digestion, and detoxify the body.

Beyond the physical aspects of asana, yoga is a great tool for training your mind and your breath, and for improving overall health. This is where you begin practicing your meditation in movement as well as connecting the meditation on the cushion with the meditation of practical living. Yoga can help you open the body physically and emotionally, help you sleep better, and even improve your mood.

Effects of Asana

The practice of asana affects the following aspects or planes of the human being:

- Physical (blood circulation, inner organs, glands, muscles, joints, and nervous system)
- Psychological (developing emotional balance and stability, harmony)
- Mental (improving ability to concentrate, memory)
- Consciousness (purifying and clarifying consciousness/awareness)

Asana means to take a seat or a posture. In Patanjali's sutras, the text that most yogis study and refer to, asana is referenced mainly in one place: *Sthira sukham asanam*, which means "steady comfortable posture," or "steady and comfortable should be the posture." Patanjali is probably referring to the asana in which one sits to meditate. Today, the word *asana* is generally used to describe physical postures of yoga exercise. This is not to say that the physical yoga exercise should not be practiced or valued, but is more of a reminder that the asana practice is not the ultimate goal.

Though yoga has existed for thousands of years, most of the asana practice we know today was developed more recently.

Vinyasa

This practice uses attention to breath to guide your flow in and out of poses. *Vinyasa* literally means "to place in a certain way." The word is most commonly used to describe a flow practice, thus the class title "vinyasa flow."

In vinyasa practice, the breath initiates the movement. Working on having the movement span the whole duration of the breath, we use ujjayi breath to help slow down and control the breath to match the length of the movement. This is especially useful in longer transitions, such as coming down from warrior to chaturanga.

Moving with Breath Helps to Remove Stagnation

- While inhaling, you open up and expand (example: upward dog).
- While exhaling, you fold down or in, contracting (example: downward dog).

Finding Your Limit

"You cannot step into the same river twice," Heraclitus said. You cannot step into the same body twice, either. Every day is new. Some days I feel like I can jump into some crazy poses, and in others even the most basic poses seem like a huge task. This could be for many reasons, but what matters is that we respect our body, wherever it may be. This is the first rule for a sustainable practice, which leads to a sustainable life.

Find the edge when you practice. This is the play between putting in effort to go deeper, and respecting the signals that say you've done enough. If you are the type that always pushes hard, consider taking it a bit slower, and if you tend to have an edge that is 60 percent of what you can do, try going to 80 percent.

While in a pose, stay calm, breathe deeply, and practice acceptance of where you are and where your edge is; this will allow the process of moving deeper to be gradual, safe, and appropriate for what your body can do in the moment.

Tips for Knowing Your Limit and How Far to Go

- Be alert. Observe the present moment.
- Go to the place just before pain; back off if pain is there.
- Some discomfort is fine and normal. Breathe into it.

- Move in a fresh way, as if it is your first time practicing; don't let the practice become mechanical.

- Explore breath as an indicator; notice when it becomes rapid or shallow and back off to where you can breathe smoothly.

- Move with steady, smooth, graceful movements, like in a dance.

Body Alignment

Before we do any yoga movements, we need to learn the most basic and fundamental yoga pose: *tadasana* (mountain pose). This is a simple standing pose that, when observed well, can reveal many lifelong conditions in the body. (**figs. 1–2**)

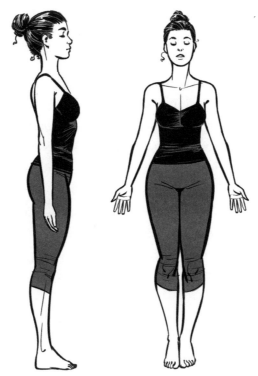

Figures 1–2, Mountain Pose side and front views (left to right)

The first time I had someone observe my body and mark the imbalances he saw in my posture, I was shocked. Some of the imbalances he found in my body were completely new to me. I had no idea that my right shoulder was a bit higher than my left. I thought I was doing so well with all the yoga I practiced.

So of course, I immediately tried adjusting myself to be balanced. It was not as easy as I thought it would be. I realized that some patterns, which I had had for many years, would take time and effort to change, until I managed to create new and healthy conditioning.

Once I got over resisting the fact that I am not perfect, I realized that accepting the imbalance would help me to fix it and get rid of it. I looked the imbalance in the eye and asked: Where is this from? As a kid, I used to carry my school bag with all its heavy books on my right shoulder.

To help carry the weight, I leaned a bit to the left, which lifted my right shoulder and compressed my left side. When I tried to imitate this movement, I noticed that my right hip lifted and the entire left side of the body became compressed. Okay, great. Now I had another thing to fix!

When we look at one imbalance, we may find another part of the body that is influenced or related to it. This is normal, as our body parts are not separate from each other.

We may even notice emotional imbalances associated with the physical imbalances. At times, an imbalance is caused by an emotional trigger—a tight chest for example.

Another imbalance I found was that my head was tilted forward. I am somewhat tall and used to be very self-conscious. I used to feel a need to hide, to beat myself up for all my imperfections.

One way I did this was to walk in what I call *slumpasasna*—or what my dad called the question mark look—which is why my head was tilted forward.

So not only was my spine twisted to one side, it was also rounded and curved in the wrong direction.

Beyond the fact that this does not look sexy, it is also unhealthy and can lead to serious back problems and pain.

Evaluating Your Posture

You can try to do this evaluation yourself in front of a mirror, but it's better to have someone else take a look at you and write down what they see. I've provided a guide to posture evaluation with diagrams below.

Your partner can write his or her findings near the body areas. It is a good idea to scan the body from the front, the back, and the sides to get a comprehensive look. (**fig. 3**)

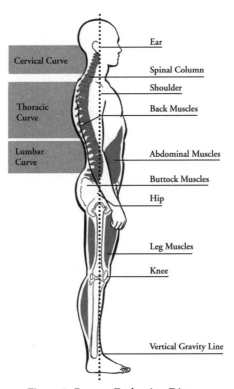

Figure 3, Posture Evaluation Diagram

Knees: Are they both facing forward?

Hips: Does one side appear higher than the other? (Your partner should place one hand on each of your hipbones to find out.)

Feet: Are they collapsed? Are the arches lifted? Is one foot turned sideways more than the other? Are they both facing more in or out rather than being parallel to each other?

Ankles: When looking from the back, are they straight and parallel to each other? Are they collapsed?

Spine: There should be three curves: one in the lower back (lumbar); one in the upper back (thoracic); and one in the neck (cervical). The curves should be visible but not overly exaggerated. For many, the lower back is either over-curved or under-curved. The mid back is sometimes flat and sometimes hunched. The neck area may have no curve, or it may be too curved in one direction. Also notice if the spine is straight or if there are any signs of scoliosis (a curvature to the left or right).

Shoulders: Are they rounded forward? Are they the same height? Are they in line with the ears and hips? Check the whole body from toes to ears. Ankles, hips, shoulders, and ears should be on the same vertical line.

Head: Is it tilted forward, back, or sideways?

General view: What else seems a bit off? There is no need to search for something that does not exist, but if you notice something, mention it. The idea is not to cure or diagnose anything; just record observations. Knowledge is the first step toward healing.

Posture Evaluation Assessment

Have a partner evaluate your posture from these positions. Write down the observations. (figs. 4–6, opposite page)

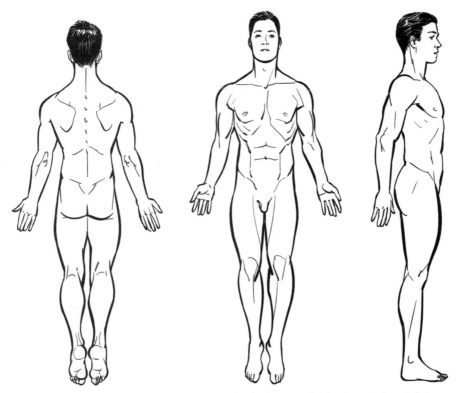

Figures 4–6, Evaluate Your Own Posture, back, front, and side views (left to right)

The Yoga Poses *(Asanas)*

Next to each pose described below, there will either be one, two, or three stars depicting the practice level necessary for it, as follows:

*Basic poses recommended for everyone and considered foundational poses, warm-up poses, or preparatory poses for intermediate and advanced poses.

**Intermediate poses which most can practice and attempt, even if it is necessary to modify them. They may require a bit more strength, flexibility, or practice.

***Advanced poses which can be practiced by students of all levels but should initially be learned with an experienced teacher and may require more practice.

These poses may include inversions, arm balances, and others that require more technical skills.

Many poses will have variations or modifications described underneath the basic pose description.

The variations are meant for students who want to try the pose in a different way, or want to deepen the pose.

Some students may find poses hard to attain due to physical limitations, difficulty focusing, or lack of technical skill.

Modifications offer the opportunity to work toward the pose, step by step, and thus help students gradually make their way into the complete pose.

Basic Alignment Principles

Hip Neutrality

Stand tall, and place the fingers of one hand on your tailbone and the fingers of the other hand on your pubic bone. Move your hips forward and back a few times, and then find the center point where both your hands, still on your pubic bone and tailbone, are at about the same height. Lift your belly in and up to support the hips to stay in this position. We call this hip neutrality. You can practice this throughout your day while standing in line, taking a walk, and to a certain degree, while sitting down. Most of us can benefit from taking the pubic bone back while seated to take away the slump from the lower back.

Shoulder Basics

Raise your arms overhead, keeping them apart. Raise the fingers high up to the sky, and then drop your shoulders down and away from the ears. Keep the palms facing each other and rotate the pinky fingers in toward one another. This will help you begin to get the shoulders to rotate out and around toward your chest as well as create space between your shoulder blades.

Now adjust the palms so that they face each other while keeping the space between the shoulder blades. This is the way we want our shoulders to be when the hands are over the head, as well as when we are in downward facing dog, handstand, and most other poses that involve the shoulders. Even in such poses as upward facing dog, where the arms are not over the head, we still want to try to create the same feeling of the shoulders rotating back and down away from the ears, as well as keep the space between the shoulder blades.

Yin and Yang

Yin and yang represent the two sides of masculine and feminine, power and softness, active and relaxed, reaching and surrendering. We contain both yin and yang within us at the same time. We may have one more emphasized than the other at different times, but even the most macho types have some feminine in them, and the girliest girls will have strength or male energy as part of them.

In most yoga classes today, there is a separation between the two aspects of yin and yang. Power classes for example, contain mostly yang energy. They will be strong, fast, and move with vigor. On the other hand, yin or restorative classes emphasize soft, long-held poses that promote surrender and release.

I love to think that every pose contains both yin and yang on different levels. Take warrior 2, for example. In this pose, there is lots of power shooting from the arms, the gaze is focused, and the legs are strong—all yang. Then the face softens, the shoulders relax, and the feet become grounded—all yin. Try to find the balance of yin and yang in all poses, and really, throughout your life.

The Warm Up

Here you will find poses that can be done at the beginning of your practice or anytime you need some release. They do not need a specific warm up, and can be done anytime. I normally start my practice with these poses (I use the warm up 1 and warm up 2 sequences) to get the energy flowing, then move on to the sun salutes and then to the standing poses. The timing of your warm up will vary according to which of the poses you choose to do and how fast or slow you move.

Basic Tips for the Warm Up

- Begin aligning *ujjayi* (victorious breath) with movement, and keep your awareness on the breath.

- Activate your *bandhas* (control centers), and focus on activating and warming up your core.

- Move steady and slowly, so you allow the body to wake up and warm up, but do not go too slow, as you do want your energy to move.

*Qi Gong Twists

Qi Gong twists (Chi gong twists) is a great warm up. I do this someimes just to move after sitting for a while. Or in the morning, when sun salutes seem to much, this is my wake-up pose. Since we tap the kidney area as we swing the arms, we awaken the lymph system, and this helps the energy flow in the body. (**fig.** 7)

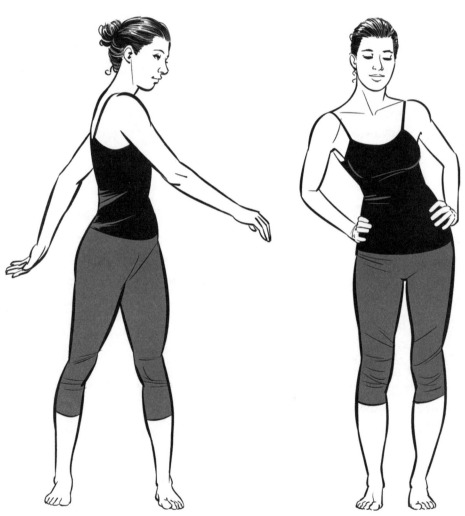

Figures 7–8, *Qi Gong* Twist and *Qi Gong* Twist Modification (hip rotations) (left to right)

Method of practice: Stand tall with your feet slightly wider than hip-width apart. Twist your shoulders and torso to the left while swinging your arms so that the left arm reaches behind you, tapping the lower back (the kidney area) and the right hand moves in front of the body toward the left lower back. Keep your shoulders relaxed.

Take the head with you so that you gaze over the left shoulder as you twist. While keeping the belly slightly lifted, keep your body movement fluid, so that you move with a sense of ease. Keep the feet steady on the floor and the knees slightly bent.

Variation: This variation is similar in the twisting action, but the hands go to different places. The left arm goes behind you; the back of the palm taps the lower back (the kidney area), and the right hand goes in front of the body, tapping the left shoulder. Take your head with you so that you gaze over the left shoulder as you twist.

Modification: A gentle variation of this is to just move the hips with the hands on the hips, as shown in the figure. (**fig. 8, opposite page**) You can do this anytime, even just as a release from prolonged sitting.

Bidalasana: Bitilasana (Cat-Cow)

The cat and cow poses are foundational warm-up poses in many yoga clases. In Doron Yoga we use delicious pose (hip rotations on all fours), as it covers more movement directions of the spine and does not take it to any extremes, but you can always choose these, if you like. (**figs. 9–10, next page**)

Method of practice: Move onto your hands and knees, hips over the knees, shoulders over the wrists, with a neutral spine. As you exhale, round the back, tuck the tailbone under, and bring the chin towards the chest. Keep the belly moving in toward the back.

As you inhale, open the chest, lift the head, drop the belly, and allow the tailbone to move back and up. With each inhale, open up, and with each exhale, round in. Take full, deep breaths. Each breath is one full movement. This is a fantastic warm up for the spine.

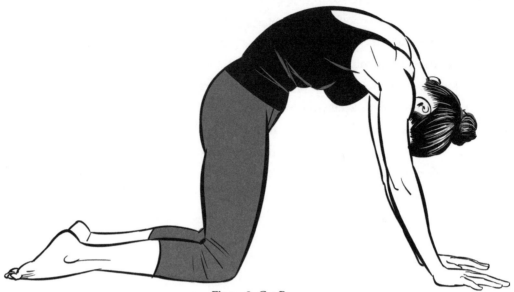

Figure 9, Cat Pose

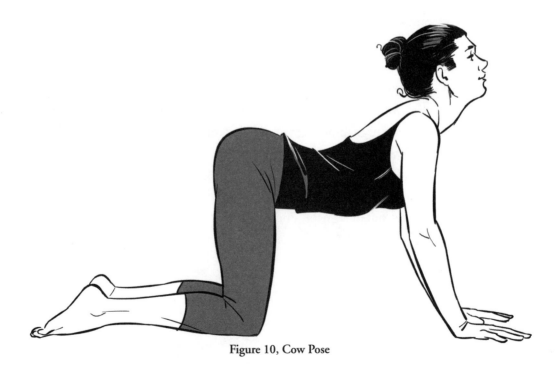

Figure 10, Cow Pose

*Hip Rotations on All Fours (Delicious Pose)

I started doing this intuitivly, as it felt great to release the spine in the morning. Some days I do this as I get up. Do this any time you need to move some energy in the body, or bring some fluidity to your joints. (**fig. 11**)

Method of practice: Come to your hands and knees, hips over the knees, shoulders over the wrists. Rotate the hips to one side while allowing the lower spine to move up and down as you rotate, thus massaging the whole lower back as well as warming up the hips. You can make the circles small or big; play around and see what feels good in your body in this specific movement. You are welcome to move further into your shoulders and elbows. I like to think of this pose as being delicious, creating fluidity in the body, moving around to warm up and release stagnation.

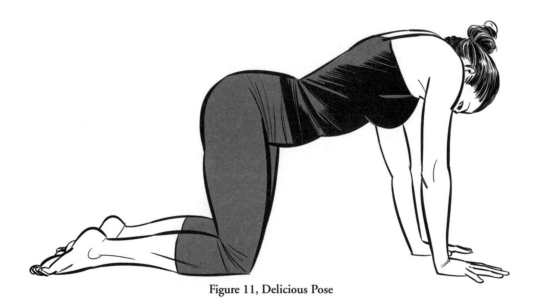

Figure 11, Delicious Pose

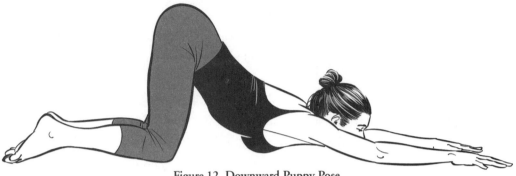

Figure 12, Downward Puppy Pose

Uttana Shishosana (Downward Puppy)

A great warm up for downward facing dog, and a good shoulder opener. Feel free to stay here longer, as it really helps melt away tension in the shoulders, chest, and upper back. (**fig. 12**)

Method of practice: From all fours, begin stretching your arms forward while keeping your hips over the knees. Relax your head down, maybe resting your forehead on the floor. If that is easy, place your chin down. Let your chest be heavy to the earth. Breathe deeply.

Head Rotations

You can do this pose anytime, preferably standing.

Method of practice: Rotate your head and neck in a full range of circular motion within your comfort zone. As the head comes forward, reach the chin toward your collarbone. Take it completely to the side, and as it goes back, try not to just drop it down but rather lengthen the neck, even if it does not go all the way back. Continue to the side and back down. For the full exercise, do five to each side, then four to each side, three to each side, two to each side, and one to each side. Respect your neck and go at a pace that feels good. It is better to start slowly.

Shoulder Rotations

You can do this pose also anytime, preferably standing. Lift both shoulders high up towards the ears and drop them back all the way while maintaining hip neutrality. Do this ten times. It helps to lift in the belly to support your hips and spine while doing this so your torso stays steady as you move your shoulders up and back. After rotating both shoulders together ten times, rotate one shoulder followed by the other shoulder for a count of ten.

Most of us have a tendency to drop the shoulders forward while driving, working on the computer, or eating, or we normally just slouch. That is why I offer rotating the shoulders back but not forward. If you find yourself uneven in the shoulders and feel the need to balance them out with a forward motion, feel free to do so, but practice this with caution.

Tri Pada Adho Mukha Svanasana (Three Legged Dog)

This is a preparation pose that helps warm up the legs and the hips. Though this pose is about lifting the leg behind you, it always feels good for me to open the hips as well, and even add some ankle rotations while the leg is in the air. (**fig. 13**)

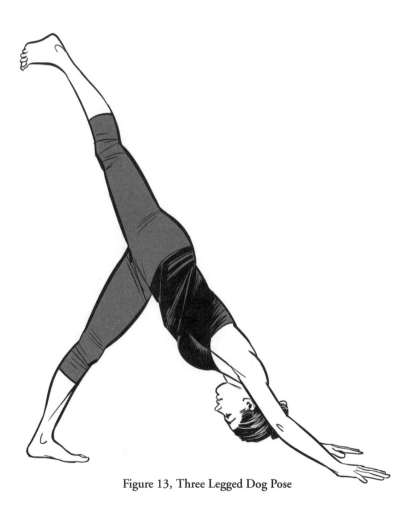

Figure 13, Three Legged Dog Pose

Method of practice: From downward facing dog, lift your right leg up toward the sky. Try to keep your hips and shoulders somewhat squared. Keep pressing your left heel to the earth.

Variation: From here, you can bend the knee and open the hips for a few breaths, so the right foot is reaching toward the left hip. I also take a few ankle rotations here as additional warm up. Then straighten the leg back behind you in preparation for knee to nose sequence.

*Knee to Nose

Bringing the knee forward helps warm up the hips in preparation for bringing the foot forward between the hands. It is also a good core warm up, especially if you do your best to bring the foot as far forward as you can while lifting it up toward the chest. The back rounds up as in cat pose to maximize the core and even warm up the back and shoulder muscles. **(fig. 14, opposite page)**

Method of practice: From tri pada adho mukha svanasana (three-legged dog), exhale as you bring your right knee forward toward the nose. Press your arm into the earth and lift in the upper back while keeping the belly lifted in (this is actually a core warm up). You will need to shift your body forward so that the shoulders come over the wrists. Inhale and take your leg back to tri pada adho mukha svanasana.

Modification: You can have the left knee on the ground while doing this movement.

*Knee to Elbow

Similar to knee to nose pose, this warms up the hips and core as well. **(fig. 15, opposite page)**

Method of practice: From tri pada adho mukha svanasana, exhale as you bring your right knee to the right side, toward your elbow or even onto the elbow if possible. You will need to shift your body forward for this. Inhale and press back to tri pada adho mukha svanasana.

Variation: Bend the elbows into chaturanga (low pushup) position with the knee still at the elbow. Inhale and press strong back to three-legged dog. This is much more challenging, but a great way to build further strength if you have an easy pushup.

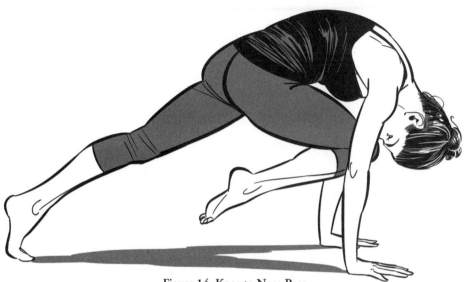

Figure 14, Knee to Nose Pose

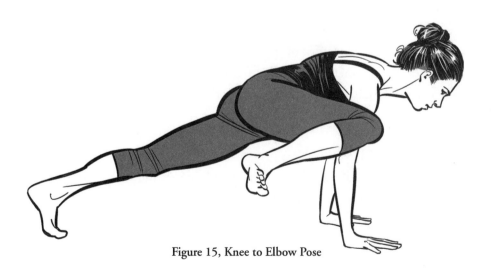

Figure 15, Knee to Elbow Pose

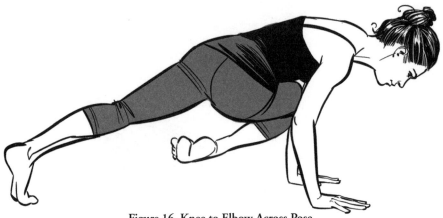
Figure 16, Knee to Elbow Across Pose

*Knee to Elbow Across

As knee to nose, and knee to elbow, this continues our warm up, with the addition of a twist in the hips as we reach the knee across. This helps activate different core muscles and further warms up the hips. (**fig. 16**)

Method of practice: From tri pada adho mukha svanasana, exhale as you bring your right knee across to the left elbow. You will need to rotate your hips and shift your body forward for this to happen. Inhale and take it back to three-legged dog.

Sun Salute Poses

The sun salutes serve to warm up the body. Traditional ashtanga classes begin with these. I add some additional warm up poses as I noticed that for most of us, not living in a tropical climate or sitting on the floor most of the day, a gentle warm up helps before we dive into these sun salutes. Practice them as a meditation. Use them to warm up the body, steady the breath and focus of the gaze (drsti), but also steady the mind, as you stay focused and present with your movements.

Basic Tips for the Sun Salutes

- Practice awareness of movement aligned with breath and with drsti. Use your bandhas (control centers) as you move.
- Be patient, especially if this is a morning practice. Allow your body to open in its own time.

- Pay attention to your transitions, they are a great opportunity to deepen the breath and practice meditation in movement. Set your focus and presence now, so it stays with you during practice.

Tadasana/Samasthiti (Mountain Pose/Equal Standing Pose)

These poses are the foundation for a healthy posture. Knowing to stand correctly in tadasana (mountain pose) will ensure that you have correct alignment in most other poses as the basic alignment of this pose keeps showing up throughout all the other poses, at times with different arm variations or a hinge at the hips. The description below explains how to do a correct tadasana. Once you understand and know this, there is no need to go through the entire process again. (**figs. 17–18**)

Tadasana and *samasthiti* (equal standing pose) are actually the same pose. Here I show tadasana classically standing, and samasthiti with hands together in front of the heart, though in a yoga class you may find that the names are used interchangeably.

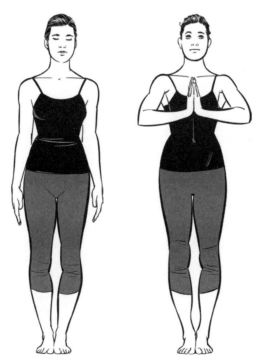

Figures 17–18, Mountain Pose/Equal Standing Pose (left to right)

Method of practice: Stand tall with the big toes and ankles touching. Lift the toes, spread them wide and activate the arches in the feet. Lower the toes while maintaining some of the arch engagement.

Move your weight slightly forward and back so that you are evenly sharing the weight between the balls of the feet and the heels.

Roll the thighs in toward each other, which might feel like a hard thing to do since when lifting the arches of the feet, the shins will tend to rotate outward. Just do your best to rotate the thighs in and work these counter rotations, which will help you root and stabilize the lower part of the body.

Find your tailbone and pubic bone and place one hand on each. Move your hips forward and back until you can find a neutral place where both hands are at about the same height, thus creating pelvic neutrality.

Lift your belly, expand your chest while filling the breath up into the shoulder blades, and rotate the shoulders down and back.

Extend your neck tall and bring the chin parallel to the floor so that the spine at the neck maintains its natural curve. Allow your hands to hang beside your body. Some like to have the hands at the heart in *namaste* (prayer), which we call here samasthiti.

Try and maintain the body as active and alive, while staying calm and relaxed at the same time. It will happen over time.

Modification: If needed, separate the feet from one another to find a steady standing pose.

Urdhva Hastasana (Raised Hands or Upward Salute)

Similar to tadasana, but with arms up over the head. This small movement reveals how open our shoulders are. Keep the arms straight here, so you can feel the energy rising all the way from your lower back (kidney area), through your shoulder blades and up to the arms. Let it feel powerful, with energy shooting out of your fingertips, while at the same time, let your shoulders relax down away from the ears. Though you maintain focus, remain calm and at ease. (**figs. 19–20, opposite page**)

Method of practice: From tadasana, rotate your palms outward and raise the arms over the head. Rotate the shoulders externally in order to create space between the shoulder blades and the neck as if wrapping the upper back in toward the chest.

Take your gaze up toward the hands and bring your hands as close together as possible while keeping the arms straight. The hands will be slightly in front of you so that as you take the head up, you might be able to see your thumbs.

Try to keep a neutral pelvis by breathing into the front and back of the body, engaging uddiyanabandha (flying up control center) and tucking the tailbone under.

Modification: If the shoulders are tight, simply keep the arms parallel to each other or as close to each other as they will go while keeping the arms straight. You can look up toward the hands, or if uncomfortable, keep the gaze forward.

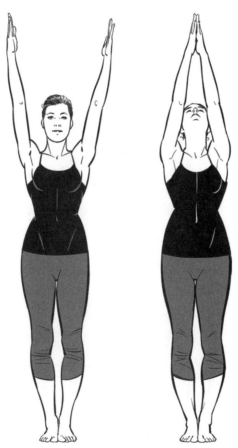

Figures 19–20, Raised Hands or Upward Salute Pose (left to right)

Uttanasana (Standing Forward Fold)

Though a part of the sun salutes and warm up 2, this pose may feel stiff for some at first. Please make sure to bend the knees as much as needed so that there is no pain in the back. Hamstring (back of the leg) stretch is fine. The legs, as well as the muscles connecting the legs and back will open and release. (**fig. 21**)

Method of practice: From urdhva hastasana (raised hands), hinge at the hips and fold forward. Place the hands beside the feet or wherever they can reach. Feel the belly slightly lifting simply by breathing into the back of the body. Press evenly into all parts of your feet as you lengthen the spine down toward the earth and relax the head and neck.

Modifications: Take the feet slightly apart and bend the knees as deeply as needed to release the hamstrings and prevent any tension in the lower back. If the hands do not reach the floor, keep reaching them in that direction.

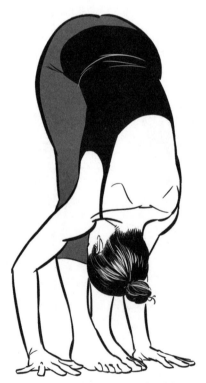

Figure 21, Standing Forward Fold Pose

*Uttanasana (Standing Forward Fold Holding Elbows)

Similar to uttanasana, except we normally hold this forward fold longer with the feet wider apart. You can always do this with knees bent to release the back. Over time, straighten the legs. This is a great pose to hold for longer durations—from ten breaths to five minutes. Doing this pose daily will prove great results for those of us with tight hamstrings (back of the thighs). (**fig. 22**)

Method of practice: Same as uttanasana, but with feet shoulder width apart and the hands holding the elbows.

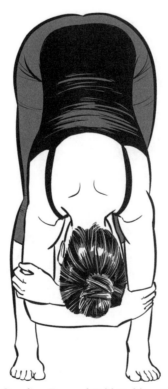

Figure 22, Standing Forward Fold Holding Elbows Pose

Pada Hastasana (Standing Forward Fold with Hands Under Feet)

This is the ashtanga version of the forward fold. There are actually two versions of this pose in ashtanga—one with holding the big toes with your peace sign fingers, and one with hands under feet. I'll explain the hands under feet here, but you can chose any variation that works for you including the holding elbows position. (**fig. 23**)

Method of practice: From tadasana (mountain pose), spread your feet shoulder width apart, inhale and lengthen the spine, and then exhale, fold forward, and bring the hands to the floor and place them under the feet. With another inhalation lengthen the spine forward, and with an exhalation surrender into the pose.

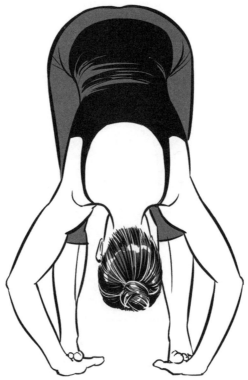

Figure 23, Standing Forward Fold with Hands Under Feet Pose

The important part of the practice in this pose is to stay a bit longer, relax the mind, and take deep exhales. You can activate the quads (front of the thighs) as this helps release the hamstrings (back of the thighs). Using your bandhas (control centers) helps create space in the spine for the forward fold and protect the back. Other that this, let gravity do the work for you. Take a deep breath and surrender into the pose.

Ardha Uttanasana (Forward Fold, Half Way Up)
The lengthening of the spine forward and half way up from the ground, serves as an opportunity to reactivate the bandhas and recreates space in the spine. (**fig. 24**)

Method of practice: From uttanasana, lengthen your spine, coming up onto the fingertips so the back is straightening forward. Lengthen the neck forward so the entire spine is long, from the tailbone to the crown of the head. Activate your bandhas and lift the kneecaps, thus engaging the legs.

Modification: Bring the hands to the shins in order to have enough room to completely lengthen the spine.

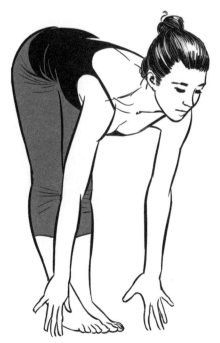

Figure 24, Forward Fold, Half Way Up Pose

Utthita Chaturanga Dandasana (Plank Pose)

Plank pose is mostly used as a transition position before lowering down to chaturanga (low push up). It can also be held for longer periods in order to strengthen the core and shoulders. (**fig. 25**)

Method of practice: From ardha uttanasana (forward fold, half way up), step one leg back and then the other. Straighten both legs, knees off the ground, and bring the hips level with the entire body so that your body is in one even plane.

Keep the neck long by reaching the head forward. Spread your fingers, pressing all ten fingers firmly into the mat, heels pressing back and shoulders over the wrists. Lift in the belly, keeping the tailbone tucked under so that you maintain one long line from the heels to the head. Micro-bend the elbows.

Modification: You can lower the knees to the ground until you are strong enough to lift the knees off the ground.

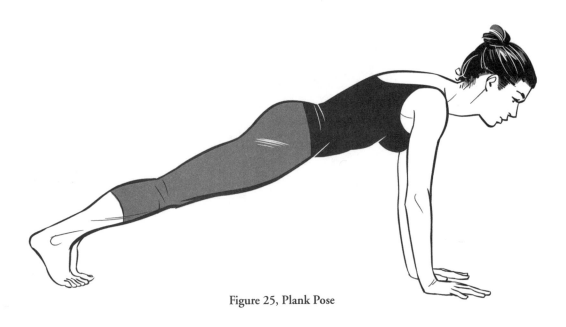

Figure 25, Plank Pose

Chaturanga Dandasana (Four Limb Staff Pose, Low Push Up)

The low push up position is a transition pose before upward facing dog. It helps tone the body and keeps us strong. For some of us this is very easy, while for some it is a long-term goal. Be patient with it, and do it correctly, even if it means knees on the ground for many years. Too many people rush into doing it with knees up, and when lowering down they collapse into the shoulders. Since we do this pose often, this can lead to shoulder injury, so go slow, and practice often. (**fig. 26**)

Method of practice: From plank pose, keep the heels reaching back, and the legs and belly activated. Slowly bend the elbows back while keeping them close to the body. Lower the body until the shoulders and elbows are at the same height and hold until you finish your exhale. Keep the shoulders rotating up and back. Keep the chest slightly open so that the gaze is forward. Try to keep the hips in line with the legs and torso.

Modification: Drop the knees and bend the elbows only an inch or to a place where you feel you can hold steady for a full breath. While lowering down, make sure your shoulders do not move forward. While bending the elbows back, keep your shoulders over the wrists.

Variation: See ashtanga pranam on the next page.

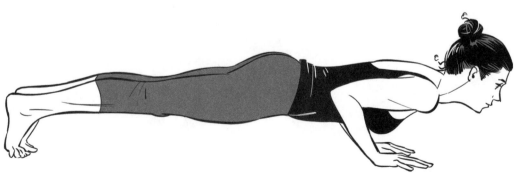

Figure 26, Four Limb Staff Pose, Low Push Up Pose

Ashtanga Pranam (Knees, Chest, Chin, or Eight Limbed Pose)

This is a classic pose in hatha yoga (physical yoga), and a great modification for chaturanga (low pushup). You may practice this as a substitute for low push up regularly or just use this at the beginning of practice until you warm up enough for the low push up position. (fig. 27)

Method of practice: Starting in plank pose, lower the knees down to the floor, shift the hips slightly back, and lower the chest in between the hands. Rest your chin on the floor. Your hips will be high up toward the sky. Keep the elbows close into the body, shoulders moving back and palms pressing into the earth. Over time, try to keep the shoulders closer to the wrists, rather than very far forward.

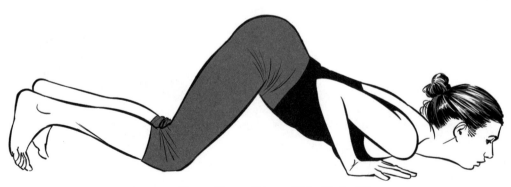

Figure 27, Knees, Chest, Chin, or Eight Limbed Pose

*Urdhva Mukha Svanasana (Upward Facing Dog)

This may be your first backbend of the practice, so go easy at first and slowly allow yourself to take the full expression of the pose. It is easy to forget to breathe here—try to take a deep inhale as you open the chest. (**fig. 28**)

Method of practice: From chaturanga (low push up*)*, inhale as you slide forward and up, extending the back and chest. Press the tops of the feet into the earth, activate and lift the legs, and nearly straighten the arms. Keep a micro-bend in the elbows. The chest keeps moving forward to lengthen the lower back, as well as lifts toward the sky. The gaze is slightly up to help lengthen the neck, but do not overarch the neck as that will lead to compression. Reach the crown of the head up.

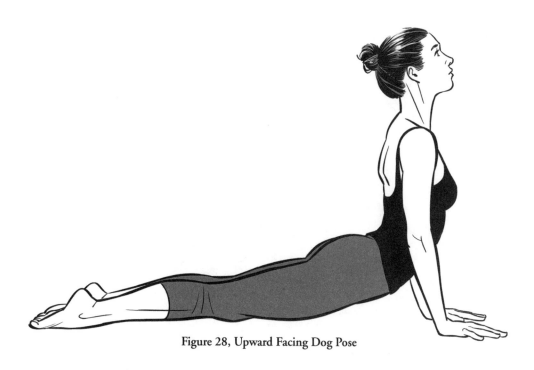

Figure 28, Upward Facing Dog Pose

Adho Mukha Svanasana (Downward Facing Dog)

Downward facing dog helps stretch the back of the legs, the shoulders, and over time lengthen the back. At first this pose may seem very difficult but eventually it becomes a resting pose. It is practiced every time we take a vinyasa, and as part of the warm ups as well as the sun salutes. (**fig. 29**)

Method of practice: From urdhva mukha svanasana (upward facing dog), exhale as you lift the hips and shift them back, rolling over the toes and pressing into your hands. The distance between your hands and feet should be the same distance they would be from each other in plank pose. Keep the feet hip-width apart and work toward straightening the legs back and reaching the heels toward the earth. Hips reach up and back creating more space for the back to lengthen. Hands root into the earth so that all your knuckles are pressing into the mat. Try to maintain the space between the shoulder blades by slightly rotating the shoulders towards the chest. After you rotate the shoulders, lift them to the same level as your torso. Lengthen the front and back of body, feeling your belly lift to help lengthen the lower back. Let your head hang between your hands, and of course breathe.

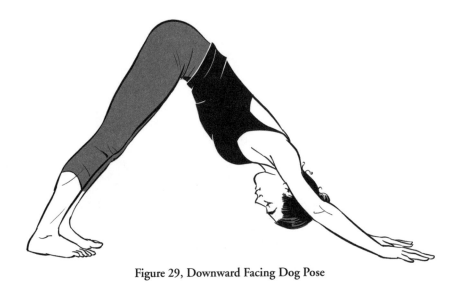

Figure 29, Downward Facing Dog Pose

Standing Poses

Standing poses are great for preparing for some of the more challenging poses. They offer the opportunity to stretch most of the body in a safe manner and continue to warm the body up.

Standing poses help steady and focus the mind, and if done with awareness, they encourage correct alignment and awaken the flow of energy. Some standing poses can be part of the sun salutes.

Basic Tips for Practicing Standing Poses

- Be aware of the tendency to be sloppy in standing poses, as they feel more familiar compared to backbends or seated poses.

- Stay grounded through the feet, and engage the legs. Keep knees micro-bent to protect the joints and activate the quads. Use inhales to create space and length and exhales to allow a deepening of the pose.

- The pelvic floor—mulabandha (root control center)—should be activated to help create length in the spine and stability in the pose. Keep the bandhas (control centers) active, both in the transitions as well as in the poses. Begin with the bandhas (control centers), and then lengthen in the lower back to allow the pelvis to lift and move over the femur heads to create proper alignment.

- Pay attention to transitions.

Pada Hastasana (Standing Forward Fold)

Forward folding is a good way to stretch the back of the legs. For many of us, doing so standing is safer and less stressful than in a seated position. Allow yourself time to release into the pose. This a great pose to be in for longer holds, and is especailly helpful for runners, skiers, cyclists etc. (**figs. 30–31**)

Method of practice: From samasthiti, inhale and lengthen the spine, exhale and forward fold. Place the hands under the feet, lengthen once more and then forward fold. Like most poses stay for five breaths, but if you would like to achive quicker results in releasing your hamstrings, stay at least ten breaths, and up to five minutes.

Modification: If it is hard to reach or it is too much pressure on the hamstrings (back of the thighs), or the back, bend the knees as much as needed. You can also hold the toes instead as that is a bit easier to reach. If all this is too much, simply stay with the uttanasana modification of holding the elbows as you forward fold.

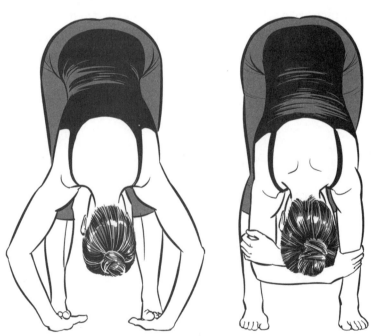

Figures 30–31, Standing Forward Fold Pose and
Standing Forward Fold Modification Pose (left to right)

*Utkatasana (Awkward Chair/Fierce Pose)

This pose is good for strengthening the quads (front of the thighs). It is practiced either as a transition for one breath in sun salute B, or at times practiced as a longer held pose. You can hold it for a few breaths longer anytime you take it for a breath. (**fig. 32**)

Method of practice: Bend the knees, and with an inhalation, raise the hands over the head. The hands can be apart or, if able, work toward bringing them together.

Try to keep your pelvis neutral (the tendency is to stick the buttocks out). Tuck the tailbone down slightly. Keep lifting the arms, reaching the fingers upward.

Open the chest and breathe into the front and back of the body. This pose can be challenging or awkward, so I like to practice smiling in this pose (thus I renamed it "happy pose"). The gaze can be forward or, eventually, up toward the hands.

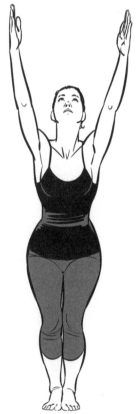

Figure 32, Awkward Chair/Fierce Pose

Anjaneyasana (Low Lunge)

Low lunge is a safe way to stretch the hip flexors—or the upper part of the leg that connects with the hips. These muscles help us move our legs, such as when we walk or run. Low lunge also serves as a preparation for backbends, since most backbends require the hinging of the hips in the same way. You can practice this anytime, as part of the warm up, preparation for splits, or before backbends. Both of these low lunge variations can be held for longer to achieve greater benefit, and quicker release of the hips and quads, including the psoas muscle. (**fig. 33**)

Method of practice: From downward dog position, lift the left leg up into the sky, coming up onto the toes of the right foot, bend your left knee and start to bring it toward your chest while lifting in the belly and shifting your shoulders forward to the wrists. Land the foot between the hands. If the foot does not reach there, help yourself with the left hand and move the foot forward between the hands.

Lower the right knee to the floor or a blanket and lift your hands onto your left thigh. Lengthen the spine as you sink forward into the left knee. You will feel the stretch in the front right thigh.

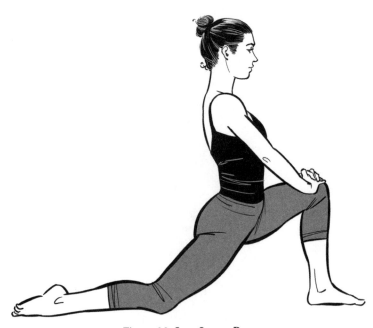

Figure 33, Low Lunge Pose

Variation: Quad stretch. Bend the right knee, and lift the leg up toward your hip. If possible, hold your foot with your hand and begin to move it forward, eventually turning the fingers in the same direction as the toes. This will deepen the stretch and move it from the hip flexors (thigh, closer to the hips), to more of a quad (center thigh) stretch. (**fig. 34**)

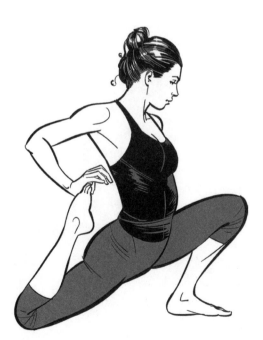

Figure 34, Low Lunge Variation (quad stretch)

Anjaneyasana (High Lunge/Crescent)

The high lunge is a great pose to strengthen the legs and stretch the hips. It is also a great preparation for the warrior 1, as here the back foot is up, and thus easier to have the hips square forward. (**fig. 35**)

Method of practice: Step the right foot forward while the back heel stays up. Reach up with a long spine supported by your bandhas (control centers) and then lift the arms up towards the sky. Keep the lift in the belly, and tuck the tailbone down creating a neutral spine. Keep reaching the fingers towards the sky while pressing the shoulders into the back and away from the ears. Sink into the hips, keeping the back leg very active, with the back heel reaching far back. The front knee should not go beyond the ankle. If you are bending deeply and you find your front knee moving past the ankle, scoot the front foot forward so the ankle is right below the knee. Repeat on the other side.

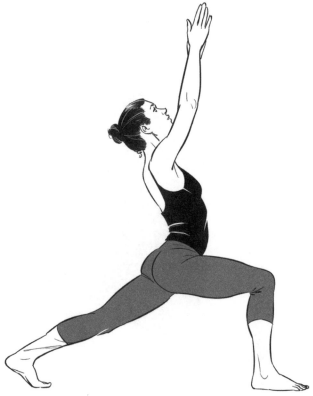

Figure 35, High Lunge/Crescent Pose

*Virabhadrasana Ka (Warrior 1)

Warrior 1 is a powerful pose practiced by many schools of yoga. Feel the energy of the arms reaching up, extending the spine with them, while keeping strong grounded legs. Though it appears early on in ashtanga and vinyasa classes, doing this pose correctly is not an easy task. Work on squaring your hips forward, but do not worry if you are not able to do so. If needed, you can always do high lunge instead. It is the process that counts. **(fig. 36)**

Method of practice: From downward dog, bring your left foot forward between the hands; spin your right heel down 45 degrees. Keeping the left knee bent at 90 degrees, lift the arms and strengthen the spine. Keep your hips squared towards the front of the mat. If this is too much, you can have less of a bend in the front knee; just make sure not to take the knee beyond the ankle.

Keep the fingers reaching high up towards the sky and gaze up towards the hands while the shoulders reach down away from the ears. Lift in the belly and keep the legs strong.

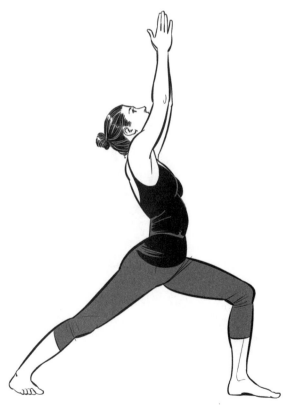

Figure 36, Warrior 1 Pose

Twisted Warrior 1

I started doing this variation as I noticed I was needing a twist early on to release the mattress from my spine (when practicing in the morning). It should feel good, just make sure to breathe while twisting. (**fig. 37**)

Method of practice: From warrior 1 pose, bring your right hand onto the left thigh, and begin to twist to the left. Place your left hand behind you wherever it reaches. Take your drsti (gaze) with your twist, to help you go deeper.

With every inhalation, lengthen the spine, and with each exhalation, deepen the twist.

Modification: You can keep the back heel up, similar to lunge pose. This helps the hips align more forward and is especially important if you feel any pressure on the back knee.

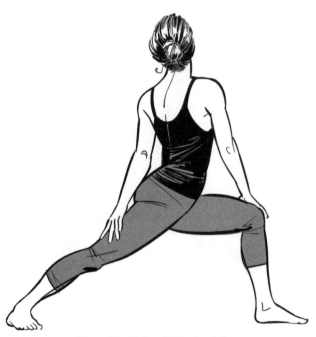

Figure 37, Twisted Warrior 1 Pose

*Humble Warrior (Surya B2)

Humble warrior warms up the shoulders and hips while forward folding in the warrior, thus also building strength in the legs. (**fig. 38**)

Method of practice: From warrior 1 pose, take the hands behind your back and clasp the fingers. Inhale, lengthen the spine and exhale, fold forward with the arms going over the head towards the floor. Go toward your thigh, or if possible, take the head and shoulder to the inside of your thigh. Keep the back leg strong, and make sure your front knee does not go beyond the ankle. Stay for five breaths and then come back up to the warrior 1 pose, and with an exhalation, lower down and take your *vinyasa*.

Modification: Hold a strap or a towel between the hands if the shoulders are tight.

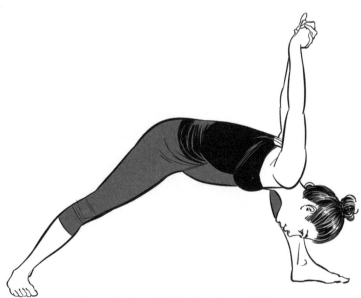

Figure 38, Humble Warrior (Surya B2) Pose

Eagle Arms Warrior (Surya B3)

Surya B3 has two parts to it. The first part opens the shoulders and the second part (lizard) opens the hips. Similar to B2, but a deeper hip opener, and a shoulder strech in the opposite direction that includes a backbend (vs. forward fold in Surya B2). This backbend can be intense, so go slow, and make sure you maintain a steady breath. It is a fantastic warm up for the deeper backbends that follow. (**fig. 39**)

Method of practice: From warrior 1, clasp your left arm under the right arm (eagle arms), engage your bandhas, keep the hips low, and begin lifting the arms up and back. This will stretch the shoulders and back. Deepen your backbend while lifting from the chest, to prevent collapsing into the lower back.

Stay for five breaths and then return to warrior 1.

Modification: When wrapping the arms, hold on to what you can reach. The hands may touch or not, maybe you reach a thumb. Whatever you can do is great.

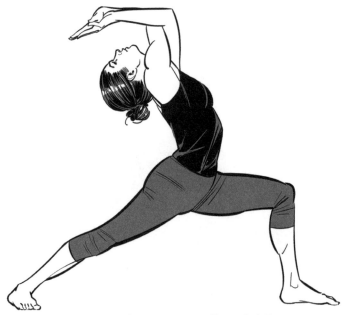

Figure 39, Eagle Arms Warrior (Surya B3) Pose

*Utthana Pristhasana (Lizard Pose)

Lizard takes us deeper into the hips, really opening up and releasing tension, as well as preparing for more challenging poses. Lizard can be very intense for some of us, so be gentle. Go just as far as you can and hold for ten breaths. Staying longer really allows the hips to relax and open. Lizard is a different stretch than pigeon, and both of these poses are important, so make sure to practice each of them according to the instructions. **(fig. 40)**

Method of practice: From warrior 1, bring both hands down to the floor to the inside of the front leg. Lower to your forearms and allow your knee to open to the side. This is actually a hip opener, but we normally practice it as part of surya B3 (sun salute B3). If this is easy, keep moving your arms forward to deepen the stretch.

Modification: Place your forearms on a block, or even stay up on your hands. Allow your hips to open gradually and go further only when it feels fine for you.

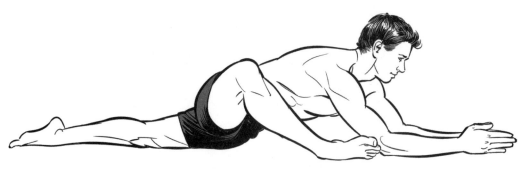

Figure 40, Lizard Pose

Virabhadrasana Kha (Warrior 2)

Warrior 2 is a pose that embodies the power of the body with the clarity of mind. This is a great pose to balance power with softness—yang with yin. Feel the energy in the body and focus the mind. A great pose to hold for a bit longer, ten breaths or more if you can. **(fig. 41)**

Method of practice: Coming up to warrior 1 with the left foot forward, slowly open to warrior 2 by bringing your left arm forward and your right arm back, parallel to the floor. At the same time, open the chest and open the hips to the sides. Both thighs should rotate externally in this pose.

Keep the left knee over the ankle; it may have a tendency to drop inward. Reach the arms away from your center as if there is a fire hose shooting water through your fingertips. Keep the power and energy in the arms but relax the shoulders.

Keep the spine long and perpendicular to the floor. Use your bandhas (power centers) to help you stay tall, and keep the tailbone tucked under so that you do not overarch in the lower back. Keep the back leg strong and root into the outer edge of the back foot. Gaze forward over the front middle fingers with intention and softness at the same time. Stay focused and calm.

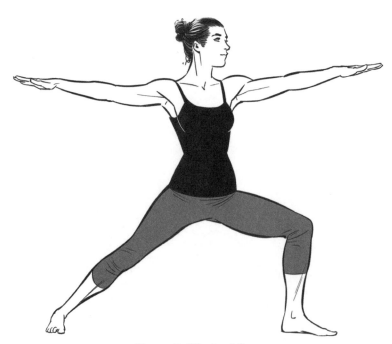

Figure 41, Warrior 2 Pose

*Viparita Virabhadrasana Kha (Reverse Warrior 2)

The reverse warrior 2 is a side stretch. There are not many of these in ashtanga classes, so I added it here as a regular practice. (fig. 42)

Method of practice: From warrior 2, inhale and rotate your left palm up to the sky. Drop your right arm to the right leg and take the left arm up and back to create a stretch in the side of the body.

Lengthen both sides of the spine and try to keep your hips neutral. There is a tendency to let the buttocks stick out; use your bandhas (power centers) to prevent this from happening. Keep the front knee bending and let your gaze follow your hand. Enjoy for three to five breaths.

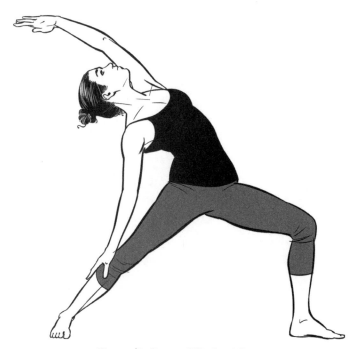

Figure 42, Reverse Warrior 2 Pose

Trikonasana (Triangle)

Triangle is a yoga classic and a good warm up for all levels. **(fig. 43)**

Method of practice: From warrior 2, straighten your front leg (without locking the knee joint), and reach forward with your left arm and torso as far as you can go. Now, lower your left arm to the left leg or even floor if possible. (The ashtanga tradition recommends holding the big toe with your peace sign fingers, if possible).

Take the right arm up to the sky and bring your gaze up towards the right hand. Keep your chin slightly tucked into the chest so that you turn the head with a long neck. Both legs remain straight and active.

Modifications: If there is discomfort in the neck, look to the side or down to the floor. Bend a bit with the front knee and activate the front of the leg to protect the knee.

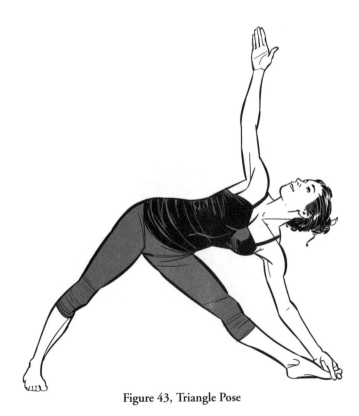

Figure 43, Triangle Pose

Utthita Parsvakonasana (Extended Side Angle)

Similar to triangle, extended side angle is a classic warm up with the hips externally rotating. (figs. 44–45)

Method of practice: From reverse warrior 2, come forward and place your left hand on the floor outside the left leg. Place the back arm alongside the body facing up, and keeping the rotation of the shoulder, bring the arm over the head so that it creates one long line from your back heel through the back leg and side of the torso through the arm.

Press firmly into the outer edge of the back foot. Press your left arm against the left leg to help you open the chest towards the sky. Take the gaze up towards the sky.

Modification: If taking the hand to the floor causes the chest to collapse, come up and bring your front forearm onto the front thigh. Press the forearm down and lift the body so that you are not collapsing into the thigh.

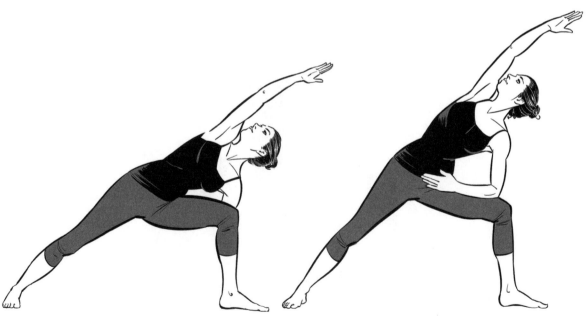

Figures 44–45, Extended Side Angle Pose and Extended Side Angle Pose Modification (left to right)

Prasarita Padottanasana A (Wide Legs Forward Fold A)

Wide legs forward fold offers a good stretch for the legs, a release for the spine, and a chance to surrender to gravity. (**fig. 46**)

Method of practice: Step the feet about four feet apart with both feet parallel to the outer edge of the mat. Place your hands on the hips. Inhale, lengthen the spine and with an exhalation, fold forward and bring your hands to the floor.

Place the hands shoulder-width apart and bend the elbows straight back, creating an arm position as you would in chaturanga (low push up). Press the heels of the hands into the floor to help the head reach towards the earth. Keep the legs straight and strong with the thighs active.

Modifications: If you feel very tight and have a hard time folding forward, take the feet farther apart. If your head reaches the floor and it is too easy, bring your feet closer together.

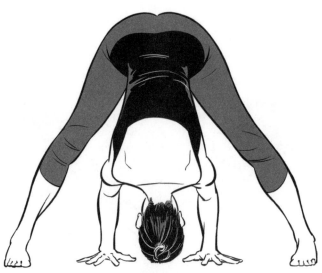

Figure 46, Wide Legs Forward Fold A Pose

Prasarita Padottanasana C (Wide Legs Forward Fold C)

This variation of the wide legs forward folds adds a shoulder stretch and some extra weight as the arms reach over the head. Stay here a bit longer. Ten breaths are great. (**fig. 47**)

Method of practice: Set your legs as in prasarita A (wide legs forward fold) and clasp the hands behind your back. Inhale and lengthen the spine; exhale and fold forward. Take the hands over the head towards the floor. Keep the legs strong and active. Breathe and try to lengthen the spine while the head reaches the floor.

Modification: If you have a hard time clasping your hands behind the back or reaching them forward, you can use a strap or a towel, holding one end in each hand as wide as feels comfortable. This will create more space in your shoulders and the ability to take the hands forward so that gravity can help you stretch deeper.

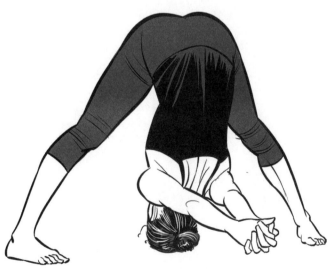

Figure 47, Wide Legs Forward Fold C Pose

Parsvottanasana (Pyramid Pose)

Pyramid pose is good for stretching your hamstrings (back of the legs) while standing. If you are struggling in this pose and need some mental help, consider repeating this mantra (chant): "I love you, hamstrings." Just repeat it over and over. No need to fight the body where it is tight, but rather send the tight areas loving energy. (**fig. 48**)

Method of practice: Step your right foot back about one leg distance from your left foot with the back foot at a 45-degree angle. Keep the hips squared forward and take reverse prayer behind the back (palms facing each other, fingers towards the head). Inhale and lengthen your spine.

Keeping the front leg straight, exhale and fold over. Keep a micro-bend in the front leg to protect the knee. With every inhalation, lengthen the spine from the place you feel it rounding the most and with every exhalation, surrender into the pose. Eventually your gaze will be towards the toes of the front foot.

Modifications: If the arm position is not available, simply hold the elbows behind the back or keep the hands on the hips to help keep the hips squared. If there is any discomfort in the knee, or if you have a knee injury, bend the front knee a bit and keep the front thigh activated.

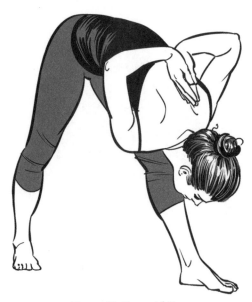

Figure 48, Pyramid Pose

Parivrtta Trikonasana (Revolved Triangle Pose)

The revolved triangle is much harder than the triangle pose, so use a block when needed, and be patient. I could not reach the floor when I started, and now I go across with the hand flat on the ground. Practice with a smile, and with time it will happen. **(fig. 49)**

Method of practice: Step your left foot back about one leg distance from your right foot with the back foot at a 45-degree angle. Keep the hips squared forward. Reach the left arm up and begin moving it forward and down towards the outside of the right foot.

Reengage your bandha, lengthen the spine, and begin to rotate the chest up as the right hand reaches up to the sky. Follow the right hand with your gaze.

Modifications: Lower the left hand to a block on the inside or eventually outside of the foot. When that is easy enough, lower the hand to the inside of the foot, then to the ankle, and eventually take the full pose with the hand outside the foot.

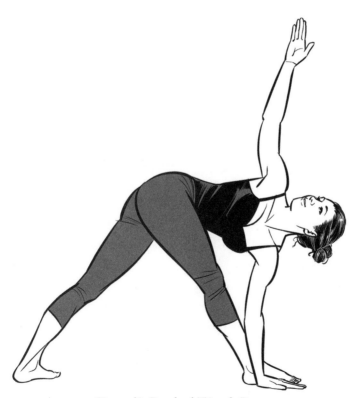

Figure 49, Revolved Triangle Pose

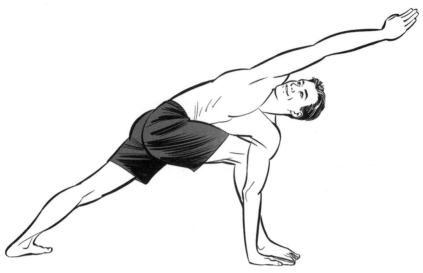

Figure 50, Revolved Side Angle Pose

Parivrtta Parsvakonasana (Revolved Side Angle Pose)

The full pose is very challenging, but luckily there are many variations for the revolved side angle. Choose the appropriate one for you. Remember that each day may be different. **(fig. 50)**

Method of practice: Step the feet as wide apart as in warrior 1. Engage your bandhas and take your left arm across and over the right knee. Try to tuck your arm so that you are reaching your armpit towards the thigh. Take the left hand to the earth, lengthen your spine, and begin to rotate your chest to the sky. Take your right arm over the head and your gaze towards the right hand or up to the sky.

Modifications: Traditionally, the gaze is towards the right hand, but you can simply look up so as not to strain in the neck or even down to release the neck and help with balance.

Most of us will need to keep the back heel up as in lunge pose rather than down as in warrior 1. **(figs. 51–52, opposite page)**

You can do this pose with the back knee on the ground. I certainly recommend at least setting up for the pose with the knee down and then, if possible, lifting it up.

You can keep the left hand to the inside of the right leg and twist from there. This makes the pose available to most people, and it is a great modification for beginners. Once you take the left hand over, you may want to place the hands in prayer position rather than opening them up if you cannot reach the left hand to the earth. The right arm can go straight to the sky rather than overhead, especially if there is any neck tension.

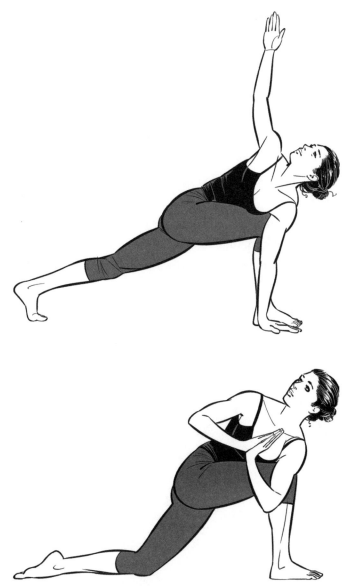

Figures 51–52, Revolved Side Angle Pose Modification (top to bottom)

Vrksasana (Tree Pose)

Tree is the most well-known standing balancing pose, and serves as a good challenge for the mind to stay focused and clear. Practice often, even without a full yoga practice, just to regain centeredness. (**fig. 53, opposite page**)

Method of practice: Standing in tadasana (mountain pose), focus your gaze on one spot that is not moving and keep your eyes soft. Let your breath deepen and soften and let your mind be calm. Shift your weight into the left foot. Grounding through the foot while continuing to spread the toes, lift your right foot up and place it on the inner thigh of the left leg. Take the right knee back so that it is in line with the standing leg. Bring your hands to your heart, find your stability, and then take the hands over the head. Slowly raise your gaze up to the sky. A steady gaze is a very crucial part of this pose. Moving your gaze will challenge your ability to stay steady.

Variation: If your hips feel open, you can bring the right foot into half lotus with the right ankle on the left thigh.

Modifications: Lift the non-standing foot to any height, from keeping the toes on the earth and leaning the heel on the ankle of the standing leg to anywhere else on the leg that feels comfortable, except for directly on the knee, especially if the knee is locked. Maintain a micro-bend in the standing leg.

Take this pose in stages. You can start with looking down and, over time, practice lifting the gaze.

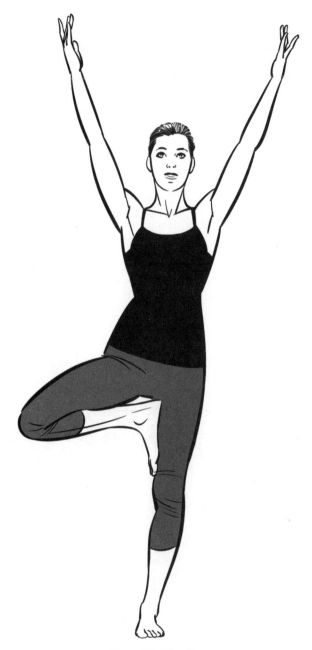

Figure 53, Tree Pose

Virabhadrasana 3 (Warrior 3)

Warrior 3 is a very challenging pose to do correctly, but you can always work towards it. Not only is it a balancing pose, but it also strengthens the glutes and standing leg. (**fig. 54**)

Method of practice: Standing on the left leg, raise your right leg back behind you as you reach the torso forward. Keep the hips over the standing leg, bandhas (control centers) engaged and back leg strong with the foot flexed. As you reach your torso forward, keep the chest open and reach the arms forward in front of you. Take your gaze towards the hands.

Modifications: Arms can be to the sides or in prayer position. There are also variations with hands clasped behind the back or alongside the body. You can keep the standing leg bent as much as you need to. Work on straightening the leg that is in the air.

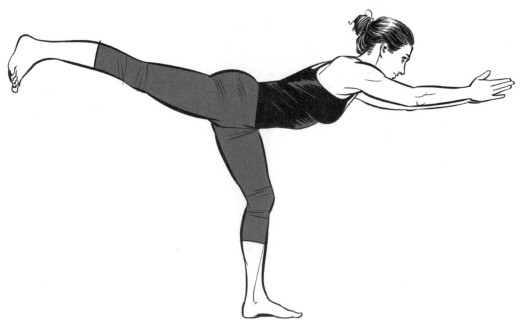

Figure 54, Warrior 3 Pose

Utthita Hasta Padangusthasana (Extended Hand to Big Toe Pose)

This is a classic ashtanga standing balancing pose. In both Doron Yoga and ashtnaga this pose comes after pyramid pose, as it requires open hamstrings, and the pyramid pose helps stretch them and prepare for this pose. This is a challenging pose, so don't get discouraged. (**figs. 55–57**)

Method of practice: This pose has three parts.

Utthita Hasta Padangusthasana A: Root your left leg into the earth, activate your bandhas (energy control centers), and focus your drsti (gaze) at one point in front of you. Lift your right leg up and reach with your "peace sign fingers" (index and middle fingers) to hold the big toe of the left leg. Optional fold over the leg. Stay for five breaths.

Utthita Hasta Padangusthasana B: From A, lift your torso up if you folded, and open your right leg to the right side. If you feel steady, try and take your gaze to your left. Stay for five breaths.

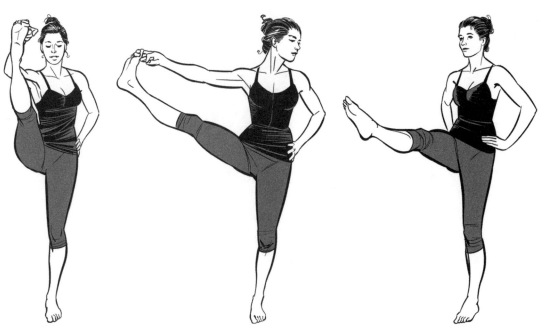

Figures 55–57, Extended Hand to Big Toe Pose (left to right)

Utthita Hasta Padangusthasana C: From B, come back to center, optional fold over your right leg for one exhale, and inhale back up. Let go of your foot, and place your hands on your hips. Keep your right leg straight and your spine tall. Try not to lean backward, even if it means your foot is just a few inches off the ground. Hold for five breaths, and release down slowly. Lucky you! One more side to go!

Modification: Since this pose is a balancing pose, but requires the hamstrings (back of the leg) to be flexible, you can do this pose with the knee bent, and hold the knee instead of the foot. You will still get all the benefits of standing on one leg, from strengthening the standing leg, to becoming more focused and stable. (**fig. 58**)

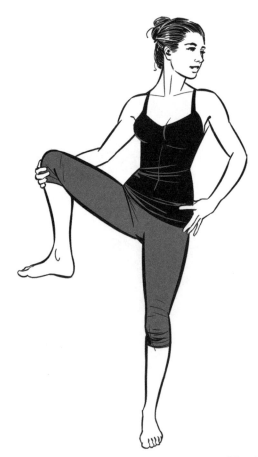

Figure 58, Extended Hand to Big Toe Pose Modification

Natarajasana (Dancer Pose)

A fun standing balancing pose, great for all. (**fig. 59**)

Method of practice: Raise your right leg behind you and hold it with your right hand. Begin tilting forward with your torso as you extend the left arm forward and the right leg back. You can move forward with your torso, but rather than going down, try to maintain an open chest, as this is a backbend on one leg.

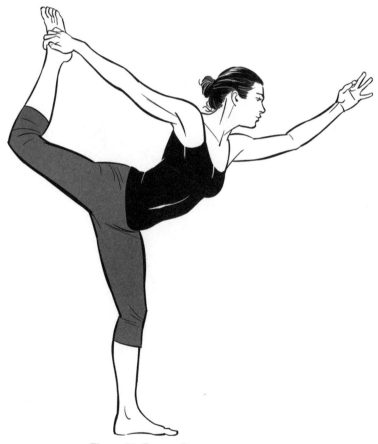

Figure 59, Dancer Pose

***Variation:* The full pose is done by taking the hands overhead and holding the foot with both hands. This is extremely advanced, but if you want to play, you can try it with a strap. This pose requires a deep opening of the entire back, the shoulders, and the hip flexors, while adding the challenge of balancing at the same time. (**fig. 60**)

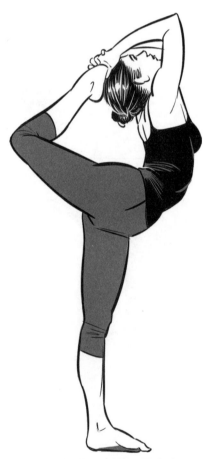

Figure 60, Dancer Pose Variation

*Preparation for the Galavasana Sage Pose/Cappuccino Pose

I like to call this pose "cappuccino" as it is easier to remember, and reminds me to sit back and down and enjoy the moment. I know I recommend not to drink cappuccinos, so you can think of it as mint tea if you rather. Whatever you do, it is a great pose as it opens the hips, strenghens the standing leg, and works on our mind to stay focused and balanced. (**fig. 61**)

Method of practice: Stand with the hands at your heart. Bring your right ankle onto your left thigh just above the knee. Keep the bandhas (power centers) activated as you begin to bend the standing knee and lower your hips down and back.

Try to keep your chest open as you bend deeper in the knee. Bend only as far as you can without letting the knee move forward beyond the ankle.

Modification: You can take the hands to the floor. You may feel a deeper stretch but will have less challenge with balancing.

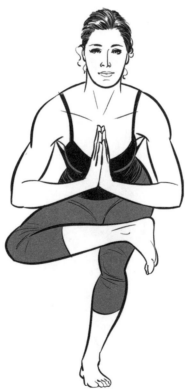

Figure 61, Preparation for the Galavasana Sage Pose/Cappuccino Pose

**Garudasana (Eagle Pose)

Eagle pose is a balancing pose that requires open hips, so take the variation that works for you, and enjoy the balancing. (**fig. 62**)

Method of practice: Shift your weight onto the left leg, lift the right leg and wrap it around the left leg. It is easier to do so, if you bend the left leg as you wrap the right. Wrap the right arm under the left arm, for eagle arms. Lower the hips back and down, so you do not shift weight onto your standing knee. Keep the arms lifted to create length in the spine and a bit of stretch in the shoulders.

Modifications: It is fine if you wrap the leg only part way. It may be that you wrap over the left thigh without tucking the foot around the calf. Your right foot may be on the ground just over the left leg. Either way is fine. It will get easier as your hips open up with the rest of the practice.

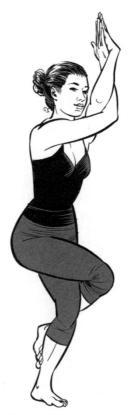

Figure 62, Eagle Pose

Ardha Chandrasana (Half-Moon Pose)

Half-moon is a balancing pose that is done as part of the external hip rotation poses such as warrior 2, triangle, and extended side angle. **(fig. 63)**

Method of practice: From triangle pose, bend slightly in the front knee (let's say the left one), and begin to shift your weight onto that leg. Lift the right leg off the ground, eventually to hip height.

Keep the hips over the standing leg, the bandhas active, and the chest opening towards the sky.

Your right hip should be stacked on top of the left or as close to stacked as your body will allow. (If the torso faces the earth, the pose becomes warrior 3.) The left hand can come to the ground; the right arm reaches up towards the sky.

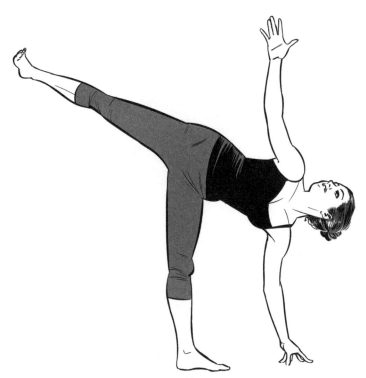

Figure 63, Half-Moon Pose

Modifications: Bend in the standing leg as much as needed, but try to keep the leg that is in the air straight. If it is hard to reach the ground with the hand, use a block.

***Variations:* Work on lifting the left hand off the ground, maybe towards the chest and balancing without its support. As an opening for the chest and shoulder, you may want to wrap the right arm behind the back towards the inner thigh. This is especially helpful when balancing without the support of the left hand. (**fig. 64**)

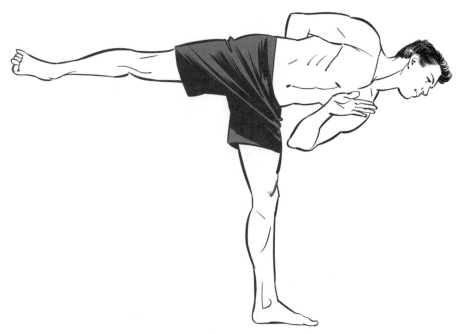

Figure 64, Half-Moon Pose Variation

Urdhva Prasarita Eka Padasana (Standing Splits)

Standing splits is a balancing pose that requires open hamstrings (back of the legs). You can always do it with a bent standing leg. Do the stretching elsewhere, and focus here on the balancing aspect of the pose. (**fig. 65**)

Method of practice: From warrior 3, lower your hands to the floor, and take the leg that is in the air, as high up to the sky as possible. Try and keep the hips square as you lift the back leg up. It may not go very far. Just do your best. The other version is to allow your hips to open, and then you may find far more space to lift the back leg. In the Doron Yoga advanced sequence we practice hopping into handstand from here. Even just the practice of hopping is good. It does not matter if you manage the handstand.

**Variation:* You can keep both hands on the ground, or take the left hand to the left ankle (standing leg) and balance here. If this still feels steady, you can try both hands to the ankle.

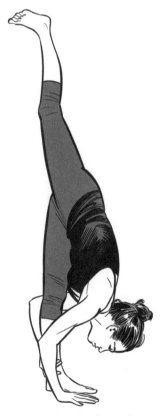

Figure 65, Standing Splits

Seated and Floor Poses

Seated and floor poses include forward bends, hip openers, and twists. Some are done seated and some reclined, lying down on the floor. In general, reclined poses are safer for beginning students, while seated poses, especially forward folds, may be challenging for those with tighter hamstrings, tight hips, and tight iliopsoas (muscles that connect the back with the upper leg) muscles. Try practicing these poses with a bit more of a yin attitude, allowing the opening to happen, rather than forcing it. I would also recommend staying in them a bit longer, at least ten breaths if you have the time. In all of these poses, focus on lengthening first, especially in the lower back, creating space for the lumbar spine, and only then deepen the pose.

Forward Folds

Forward folds open the spine, iliopsoas, hamstrings and, in some cases, the hips. All of these poses are calming and cooling and require less effort and more surrender. Since they are mostly passive, they can be held for longer durations. Breathing deeply and holding the poses a bit longer helps reduce mental and emotional fatigue. These poses are also great for balancing other more active poses such as backbends and sometimes inversions.

BASIC TIPS FOR PRACTICING FORWARD FOLDS

- Engage bandhas (control centers) to protect the lower back.
- Turn the pelvis slightly forward to allow for length in the fold. Do not go far forward until you can get the hips to tilt.
- Inhale and lengthen; exhale and move forward. Gaze slightly forward to encourage lengthening.
- Move the shoulders away from the ears and the shoulder blades away from each other.
- Rotate the thighs internally. If one foot is forward, keep toes pointing up to the sky.

- Consider keeping the quads (upper thigh muscles) engaged, as it protects the legs from injury.
- Elevate the seat on a blanket or block if any tension is in the back or bend the knees if hamstrings are very tight.

Twists

Twists are similar to the rest of seated and floor poses, though they add a few extra benefits. They tone and cleanse the internal organs, giving an internal massage that also helps with digestion. They are great for releasing the spine after any intense pose, whether it is a backbend or forward fold, or even after sitting for many hours on a chair. Reclined twists are safer than seated ones.

BASIC TIPS FOR PRACTICING TWISTS

- Sit tall with the natural curvature of the lower back. Sit on a blanket if needed.
- Use the inhalations for lengthening and the exhalations for releasing deeper into the twist. Root the sitting bones down in seated twists.
- Activate the pelvic floor and draw the belly in and up. This is both for stability and deepening. In deep twists, the coccyx should be curled in to further help with stability.
- Try to initiate the twist from the core, and then follow with the chest and upper back. Open the chest, shoulders, and neck.
- Keep the gaze moving in the direction of the twist without straining the neck and keep the head up as a continuation of the spine.

Hips

Hips are the foundation for the mobility of the body. They are a crucial part of the practice, especially in the West, where intense athletic activity and long periods of sitting on chairs and sofas cause the hips to tighten. Hip openers help with mobility of the upper and lower body. As the hips open, so do the energy centers of the lower body, centers that contain many emotional and sexual blockages. This helps us free up old patterns and releases emotional stagnation. Many back issues stem from the hips as well, so opening the hips can actually solve many back and other related problems.

Basic Tips for Practicing Hip Openers

- When hip openers are practiced as yin poses, they are most efficient. Go slowly and with patience. Never rush into hip openers.

- Inhale to lengthen the spine, and exhale deepen the pose.

- Emphasize deep long exhales to help activate the parasympathetic nervous system, which will allow for more release and opening.

- If you feel hip openers in the knees, back off. The knee is where the stretch goes when the hips are tight and we push too hard. A bit of sensation in the knee is fine, but there should not be any sharp pain.

Sukhasana (Easy Pose/Cross-Legged Pose)

A great sitting pose for anytime, including meditation. This is a good substitute for *padmasana* (lotus pose). (**fig. 66, opposite page**)

Method of practice: Sit on your mat with your legs crossed. You can sit with one leg in front of the other. Make sure you can sit comfortably with the spine straight, allowing the low back to maintain its natural arch.

If you find yourself in slumpasana, meaning you are collapsing your low back or your knees are higher than your hips, elevate your seat by sitting on the edge of blankets or a bolster. There is no limit to how high you can elevate your hips. Do your best to find a seat that allows your spine to stay long and maintain its natural curvature as well as have space for your knees drop below your hips.

*Vajrasana (Thunderbolt Pose)

A classic pose for pranayama (breath work), or as an optional position for meditation. (**fig. 67**)

Method of practice: Sit on your heels with your toes untucked and place the palms of your hands on your thighs, keeping the spine tall. Make sure there is no pressure on the knees.

Modification: If you find that the hips cannot come down to the heels or that it is uncomfortable to sit this way, place a block or a bolster lengthwise underneath your seat between the legs. Play around with the height that you need in order for your knees to be comfortable. Make sure there is no knee pain. A bit of a stretch sensation on the front of the thighs is fine.

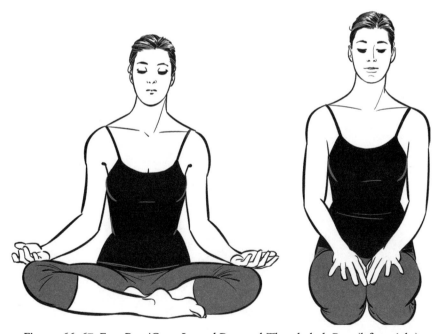

Figures 66–67, Easy Pose/Cross-Legged Pose and Thunderbolt Pose (left to right)

***Padmasana (Lotus Pose)

The classic yoga position, some say the best position for meditation, as it is very steady, even without a cushion underneath your hips. Take your time with this pose and do not force it. (fig. 68)

Method of practice: Sit in cross-legged position, bringing your right ankle onto the left thigh and the left ankle onto the right thigh, eventually allowing your toes to hang over the outsides of your thighs. Please do not force yourself into this pose, as it could hurt your knees. Be patient and practice easier hip openers such as pigeon to prepare for this first.

You can work towards full lotus by sitting with one leg in half lotus—one ankle goes over the opposite thigh, while the other leg remains as in *sukhasana* (easy pose). Stay a few breaths, and then switch the legs around. When half lotus becomes comfortable, you can start working on full lotus pose. Be patient.

Modifcation: You can work towards full lotus by sitting with one leg in half lotus.

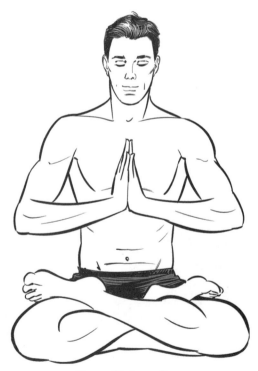

Figure 68, Lotus Pose

*Balasana (Child's Pose)

Child's pose is a great pose anytime you need a break, and a grounding pose after all inversions. (fig. 69)

Method of practice: Come onto your hands and knees with the knees hip-width apart or wider and slowly lower your hips down to your heels. Drop your chest towards the ground. Place your hands alongside the body close to the feet with palms facing up. Breathe deeply and slowly.

Variation: If you prefer, you can stretch the hands forward, palms facing down.

Modification: You can open the knees wider and let the belly drop in between the legs with the toes closer together.

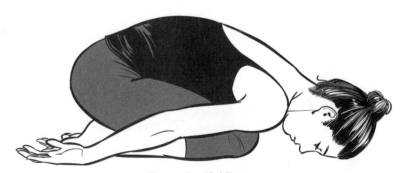

Figure 69, Child's Pose

Dandasana (Staff Pose)

This is the foundation pose for all seated forward folds. Practice this well, especially before you go into deeper seated forward folds. (**fig. 70**)

Method of practice: Sit on your mat with both legs extended in front of you. Place your hands beside your body and press into the floor to help lengthen the spine. Flex the feet, but keep the heels on the ground.

Breathe slowly into the front and back of the body to help create length in the torso. Feel your bandhas become active with your belly lifting in and up. Relax the shoulders and keep your gaze steady.

Modifications: Elevate your hips to allow for the forward rotation of the pelvis. Sit on the edge of a blanket or two. A yoga block works as well.

If you find yourself rounding a lot in your back, bend your knees. This is also a good option if you have lower back pain or knee issues.

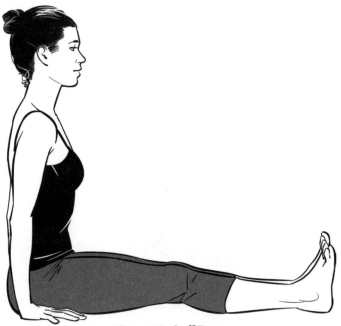

Figure 70, Staff Pose

Paschimottanasana (Seated Forward Fold)

This is the classic seated forward fold pose, taught in most yoga styles. It is a nice cooling pose that is good for stretching your hamstrings, as well as the lower back. Be gentle, as it can pull on the lower back, especially if you have any lower back pain. (**fig.** 71)

Method of practice: Sitting on your mat with your legs extended forward, lift in the belly. Keep your spine as long as possible and fold forward. Take your hands to wherever they will reach. Use your inhales to lengthen the spine, and your exhales to release and relax—especially the shoulders. Practice dandasana (staff pose) as a preparation for this pose.

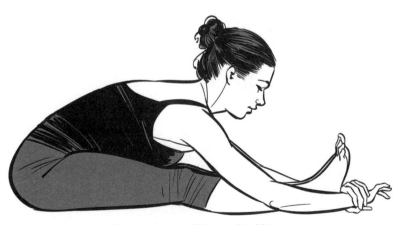

Figure 71, Seated Forward Fold Pose

Modification: If this feels tight in the hamstrings, you can bend the knees slightly as you fold forward. If you feel any tension in the lower back, elevate your seat by sitting on a block, a blanket, or bolster to create space in the lower back. Elevate your seat as much as needed, until there is no tension in the lower back. Stay for a minimum of five breaths, and up to five minutes. Do not fight the muscles but rather allow them to relax, so they feel safe to allow the stretch to happen. Try and keep your quads (upper thigh) active, to help release the hamstrings. (**fig.** 72)

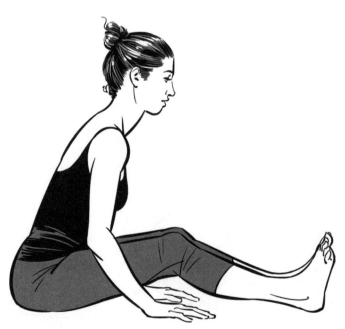

Figure 72, Seated Forward Fold Pose Modification

Janu Sirsasana A (Seated Forward Fold Over One Leg)

A nice and classic forward fold that is nice to do before paschimottanasana (seated forward fold), as there is normally less pressure on the back in this pose. (**fig. 73**)

Method of practice: From dandasana (staff pose), bend the right knee and place the right foot against the inner left thigh. Inhale, lengthen the spine, and while keeping the hips as square as possible, fold forward.

Lengthen the spine with every inhalation, extending it wherever you feel it rounding. Use your exhalations as a tool to soften and relax deeper into the pose. Keep your bandhas active to protect your lower back. Eventually, gaze towards the toes.

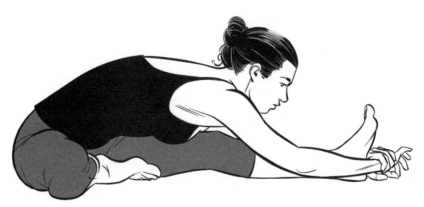

Figure 73, Seated Forward Fold Over One Leg Pose

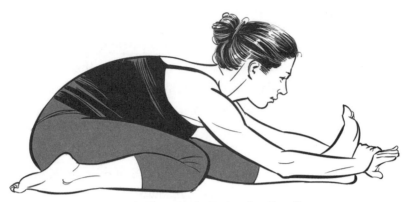

Figure 74, Three Limbs Facing One Foot Pose

**Trianga Mukha Eka Pada Paschimottanasana (Three Limbs Facing One Foot Pose)

Similar to *janu sirsasana A* (seated forward fold over one leg), but with the leg folded backward. This pose may offer additional stretching in the quads (top of the thigh), or even in the ankle or foot. To have variety, you can choose between the trianga mukha (three limbs facing one foot pose), and janu sirsasana A (seated forward fold over one leg). They give different stretches but are both forward folds. If the trianga mukha does not feel good even modified (especially in the knee), stay with the janu sirsasana A (seated forward fold over one leg) for now. (**fig. 74**)

Method of practice: Sit in dandasana and bend the right leg at the knee so that your right inner ankle is by your right hip. Try to keep the knees together while you lengthen the spine and fold forward over the left leg.

Modification: Sit on a block or blanket to help create space for the right knee as well as for ease with the left hamstring.

*Marichyasana C (Seated Twist)

A classic twist, which is a good spine release, any time in the practice or even in the middle of the day. (**fig. 75, opposite page**)

Method of practice: Sit in dandasana and bring your right knee up and your right foot to the floor about a fist distance from your left inner thigh. Keep the left leg active, left heel reaching forward, and toes turned up.

Rotate to the right side and place your right hand behind you on the floor as close to the body as feels comfortable. Bring your left upper arm to the outside of the right thigh. Use your inhale to lengthen the spine and your exhale to deepen the twist.

Modification: If the lower back is rounded, elevate your seat. If it is hard to reach the left arm to the outside of the thigh, you can hug the right knee with the left arm. (**fig. 76**)

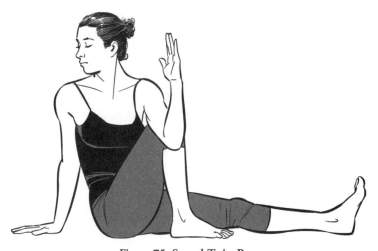

Figure 75, Seated Twist Pose

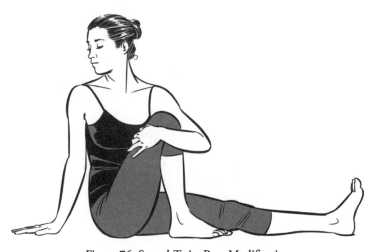

Figure 76, Seated Twist Pose Modification

Ardha Matsyendrasana (Seated Twist with the Knees Bent)

Another classic twist (and one of my favorites) that can be practiced anytime. You can always choose and exchange between this and the marichyasana C (seated twist), or if uncomfortable, you can do a supine twist instead (see p. 154). (**fig.** 77)

Method of practice: Sitting on the mat, bring the right knee up and the right foot to the floor. Bend your left knee and bring your left heel towards your right hip. Move your right foot to the outside of the left thigh.

Inhale, lengthen the spine, and begin to rotate to the right side. Take your left upper arm to the outside of the right thigh, eventually reaching your left hand to the right foot. Don't worry if it does not reach, just keep it anywhere over the right leg, even in the air. Place your right hand behind you on the floor and twist farther to the right.

Use your inhales to lengthen the spine and your exhales to deepen your twist to the right. Keep pressing the left arm against the right thigh, and if there is room, after a few breaths, move your right hand closer to the body to create more length and possibly more to the right to deepen the twist. Keep a slight bend in the right elbow to keep the right shoulder relaxed and down.

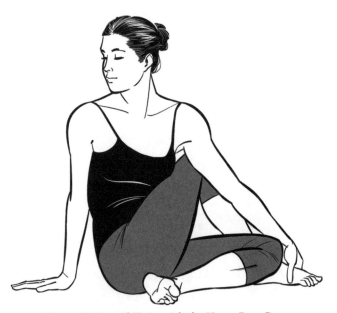

Figure 77, Seated Twist with the Knees Bent Pose

Modification: Instead of placing the left arm to the outside of the right thigh, consider wrapping the left arm around the right knee. If your lower back is rounded, sit on a block. (**fig. 78**)

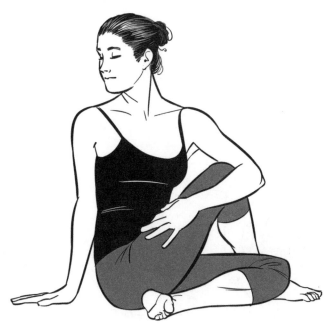

Figure 78, Seated Twist with the Knees Bent Pose Modification

Baddha Konasana (Bound Angle Pose)

A classic hip opener that can be practiced anytime, even beyond your asana (yoga poses) practice (such as reading a book, watching TV, observing a flower, etc.). (**fig. 79**)

Method of practice: Sitting on your mat with the legs extended forward, bend the knees and bring the soles of the feet together, bringing the heels close to the groin.

Place your hands on the feet and peel them open. With an inhalation, lengthen the spine, and with an exhalation, fold forward, keeping the belly lifted.

Modification: If, when sitting in this pose, you find it hard to straighten the back or the knees are high up off the floor, elevate your seat on a bolster, blanket, or block. I like to sit on the edge of the block and let my sit bones fall forward off the block. This allows my knees to drop more towards the sides so there is more weight pressing down to help my hips open.

Another option is simply to take the hands behind you and press the fingers against the floor. Try and use this action to help rotate your pelvis forward while keeping the spine long. (**fig. 80**)

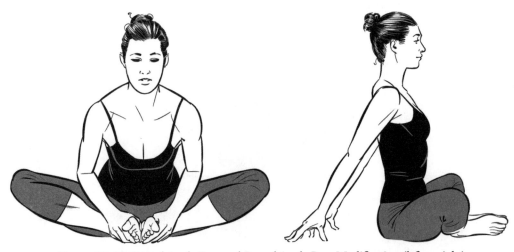

Figures 79–80, Bound Angle Pose and Bound Angle Pose Modification (left to right)

**Upavishta Konasana (Seated Wide Leg Stretch)

Like bound angle pose, this is a great pose to practice for longer durations. Sometime I place my laptop on the floor in front of me, spread my legs into the seated wide leg stretch and reach forward to work on it. Of course you can place the laptop a bit higher, depending on your level of flexibility. (**fig. 81**)

Method of practice: Sitting on your mat, keep your legs straight and spread them wide open. Inhale and lengthen the spine; exhale and fold forward, reaching the chin or chest towards the floor.

Modifications: If you find your lower back rounded, elevate your seat on a blanket, bolster, or block. You can bend your knees slightly if that makes it easier. If you find that you have to lean back in this position, place your hands behind you and slowly walk them closer to the body.

Pressing the hands or fingertips into the floor will help you tilt the pelvis forward while keeping the spine long.

Once your torso manages to come forward a third of the way, you can move your hands forward in front of you and use the hands on the floor to help you lengthen the spine with an inhale and relax your body with an exhale. Over time, you may lower down to your forearms and do the same and eventually work your way all the way down to the floor.

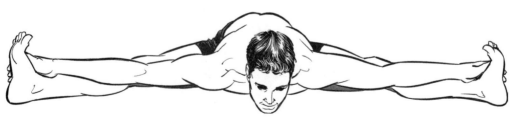

Figure 81, Seated Wide Leg Stretch Pose

***Hanumanasana (Splits Pose)

You may know this pose from dancers or other gymnastic stretches. It is very similar indeed, with just an extra emphasis on keeping the hips square. Since yoga is not about gymnastics, don't worry if you can do this or not. Simply practice, and over time your legs will release and open. Enjoy the process. (**fig. 82**)

Method of practice: From downward facing dog, bring your right foot forward between the hands, lower your left knee to the ground, and straighten the right leg. You can warm up here by folding over the right leg, or you can begin to move the leg forward for a deeper stretch if available. Eventually straighten both legs, while keeping the hips mostly facing forward. This is another great pose to hold for longer durations. From ten breaths to five minutes on each side. Do not go to the place of strong pain. Find the place where there is a nice stretching sensation, that still allows you to keep a calm and steady mind. This is a good yoga lifestyle practice.

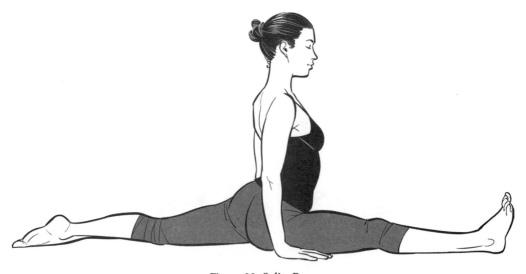

Figure 82, Splits Pose

Supta Sucirandhrasana (Reclined Thread the Needle)

This is a great foundation pose for opening the hips. It can work for all levels of students and is safe as the back is supported by the earth. Thread the needle is a great pose for those with lower back pain and especially for those suffering from sciatica. (**fig. 83**)

I highly recommend staying here for longer durations of even five minutes on each side while breathing deeply and relaxing the mind.

Method of practice: Lie down on your back, bend your knees, and place both feet on the floor. Place your right ankle over the left knee. Lift the left foot and bring the left thigh up towards the chest. Thread the right arm between your thighs and place your right hand on the upper shin. Bring your left hand from the outside of the left thigh to meet the right and clasp the hands.

Bring the left thigh as close as you can to the chest. Try to keep your lower back down on the mat. You will feel a stretch in the back of the right hip (this will stretch your IT band, the outside of the thigh). As the pose starts to become easier, work on keeping the tailbone on the ground and gently pushing your right knee away from you with the right elbow.

Modification: If you can't reach the shins, you can hold the back of the thigh. If you find your head is off the floor, you can place a block underneath the head to support it. If you have a hard time reaching your leg, you can either use a strap or place your foot on the wall (see picture). (**fig. 84**)

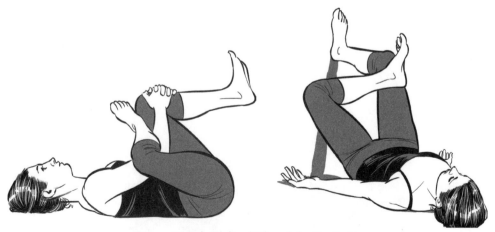

Figures 83–84, Reclined Thread the Needle Pose
and Reclined Thread the Needle Pose Modification (left to right)

Eka Pada Raj Kapotasana Prep (Pigeon Prep)

Another beautiful hip opener, that may just be the most popular one. It is similar to thread the needle, but for some this may be more intense. If so, practice thread the needle until you are ready for this. Support yourself in this pose so you are comfortable enough to stay here for longer periods. When staying five minutes, make sure to release slowly. The exit may be more intense than the pose itself. (**fig. 85**)

Method of practice: From downward dog, bring your right foot forward and place your right knee behind your right wrist. You can adjust the placement of the knee to find a spot where you feel the stretch in the hips. There should be no pain in the right knee.

Lower your left knee down and untuck the toes. Lengthen the spine and slowly lower your torso down to the floor, stretching your arms forward in front of you.

Keep the hips squared to the floor. (Try not to drop into the right hip so that both hips remain at the same height.) Keep your left leg straight behind you.

Moving the right foot up towards the head will intensify the pose, while moving it towards the hips will release some of the stretch. Another way to intensify the pose is to move the right knee more towards the right side, while moving it towards the left will make it less intense. Pigeon is best held for long periods of time. Hold for a minimum of one minute, gradually building up to five minutes.

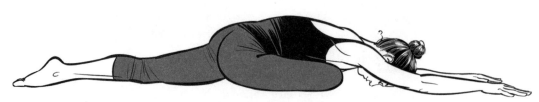

Figure 85, Pigeon Prep

Modification: Go down just as low as feels comfortable for you; you can lower to the forearms as a midpoint. Make sure there is no knee pain. If you feel a sharp pain in the bent knee, back off. (**fig. 86**)

If your right hip is off the ground, you may want to place a blanket or block underneath it for support. If you feel any pressure in the knee, please back off from the intensity. To support the knee, you may consider rolling up a small towel and placing it in the crease between the thigh and the calf behind the knee.

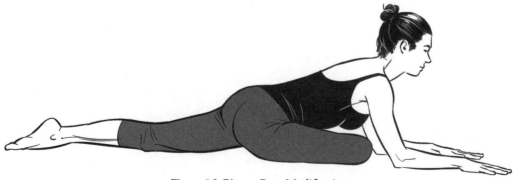

Figure 86, Pigeon Prep Modification

*Shoulder Stretch

The shoulder stretch is one of the most important stretches for the modern yogi. Most of us live life with the arms moving forward, reaching computers or other devices. This stretch really opens the shoulders and the chest in the opposite direction we normally move. Be patient with this pose. It takes time to open, and the shoulders are delicate, so stay longer, but do not push. (**fig. 87**)

Method of practice: Lie down on your belly and stretch your right arm to the side. The arm should be at the level of your nose, or just a bit higher than your shoulder level. Slowly begin to roll onto the right side over the right shoulder. Go slowly, and stop when you feel the stretch in the shoulder becoming intense.

For some it may be just a bit of a twist, keeping the left hand on the floor, pressing lightly to help deepen the stretch. If this feels fine, begin twisting further while lifting your left knee and placing your left foot on the ground or eventually both knees up.

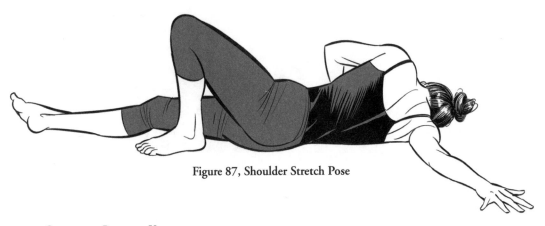

Figure 87, Shoulder Stretch Pose

Variation: For the full pose, if you are still feeling no stretch in the shoulder, take the left arm over towards the right hand and clasp hands. Do not change the placement of your right arm for the sake of connecting the hands. The goal is not to touch the hands but rather to feel the stretch in the shoulder. (**fig. 88**)

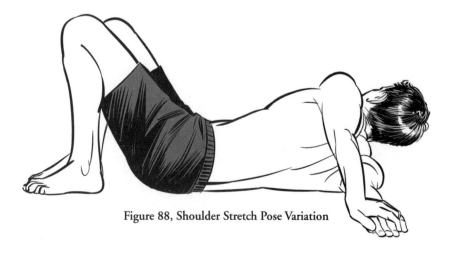

Figure 88, Shoulder Stretch Pose Variation

Jathara Parivartanasana (Supine Twist)

Supine twists are safe, help release the spine, and can be held for longer periods of time so they become restorative. They are especially good as a substitute for sitting twists when lower back pain is present. There are many variations, and you can always choose and switch them around according to what feels good for you. **(fig. 89)**

Method of practice: Lie down on your back with your feet on the ground and knees pointing up. Lift your hips and move them slightly to the left. Lower the hips and lift the knees into the chest. Take your knees over to the right. Open your left arm out to the side and place your right hand on your legs to help the legs stay down.

Take your gaze to the left. Try to keep your left shoulder close to the floor. Take deep relaxing breaths, with long exhales. Hold from thirty seconds to five minutes and switch sides.

VARIATIONS:

Jathara Parivartanasana B (Supine Twist with Eagle Legs)

If the basic supine twist is easy, try this variation. It is my all time favorite. **(fig. 90)**

Method of practice: Place the feet on the floor with the knees bent. Wrap the left leg over the right thigh, possibly even bringing the left foot to the outside of the right ankle ("eagle legs").

Keep the right foot on the floor, lift the hips and move them about a foot to the left and lower the legs to right. Open your left arm out to the side and place your right hand on your legs to help the legs stay down. Take your gaze to the left, keeping the left shoulder close to the earth.

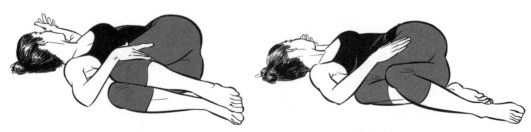

Figures 89–90, Supine Twist and Supine Twist with Eagle Legs Pose

Jathara Parivartanasana C (Supine Twist C)

Here are two more variations you can play with. All are good, see what feels best for you and change them around to get slightly different stretches. With the knees bent it is easier and will stretch more of the spine, while with straight legs you may feel more the back of the leg or even the hips. (**figs. 91–92**)

Method of practice: Keep the right leg straight, while you take the left leg over to the right. You can do this either with a straight leg or bent knee. This is sometimes known as *supta matsyendrasana* (reclined half lord of the fish pose). I offer the straight leg variation here as well as in the supine leg stretches, as it stretches more of the leg and hip than it gives a back twist, but it is useful either way.

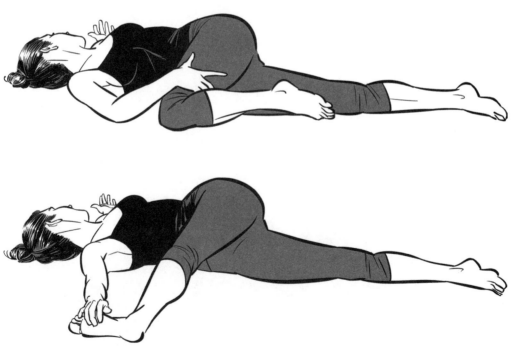

Figures 91–92, Supine Twist C Pose (top to bottom)

***Jathara Parivartanasana D (Supine Twist D)

This one requires more flexibility to get into, and may again feel more in the legs rather than the spine. Just another option to play with. Have fun! (**fig. 93**)

Method of practice: With both legs straight, twist to the right. Hold the outer edge of your left foot with your right hand. Bend the right knee and with your left hand, reach for the right foot. Take your gaze over to the left. This is a twist as well as a leg stretch.

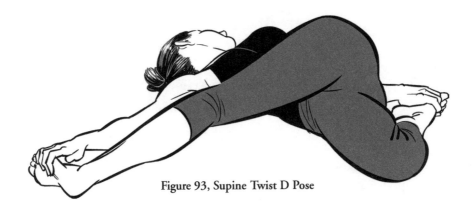

Figure 93, Supine Twist D Pose

Supta Padangusthasana (Reclined Big Toe Pose/Extended Leg Supine Stretch)

These poses are fantastic for opening up the hamstrings and stretching the legs in a safe manner. I normally add jathara parivartanasana C (**supine twist C**) as part of the sequence, after doing supta padangusthasana A and B (extended leg supine stretch A and B). This adds a nice gentle twist for the back while protecting the lower back as it is on the ground and slumping is not really an option. These poses are also beneficial for someone suffering from sciatica. (**fig. 94**)

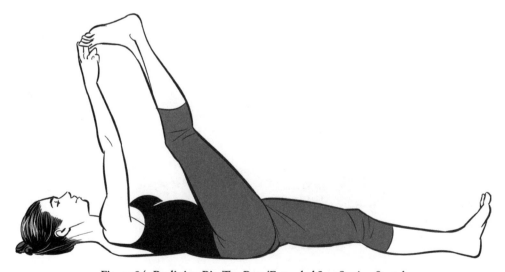

Figure 94, Reclining Big Toe Pose/Extended Leg Supine Stretch

Supta Padangusthasana A (Extended Leg Supine Stretch)

A perfect way to stretch the legs without compromising the back.

Method of practice: Lie down on your back with your legs extended in front of you and your toes facing up. Bring your right leg up and take hold of your big toe with your peace fingers. You can also simply hold the foot in any way that is comfortable for you.

Stay here and breathe deeply, watching your breath. Hold for ten deep breaths to begin with. Over time, increase the length of your hold to up to five minutes.

Supta Padangusthasana B (Extended Leg Supine Stretch to the Side)

Method of practice: From the previous pose, simply begin opening the leg to the right side, going only as far as you can, keeping the left hip mostly on the floor. Hold for five to ten breaths, eventually increasing the hold up to five minutes. Then raise the leg up to center. (**fig. 95**)

Modification: Use a strap if you cannot reach your foot. If your leg does not come up to 90 degrees, bend the knee that is on the floor, and place your foot on the ground. (**figs. 96–97, opposite page**)

This will help you bring the leg you are pulling a bit closer, so it is more efficient. Once this gets easier, you can straighten the other leg back down. When going for the opening or the twisted variations, straighten the leg with the bent knee back to the floor.

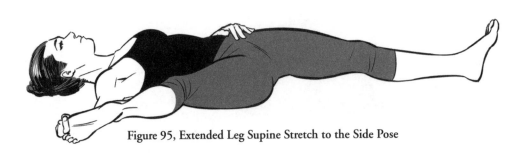

Figure 95, Extended Leg Supine Stretch to the Side Pose

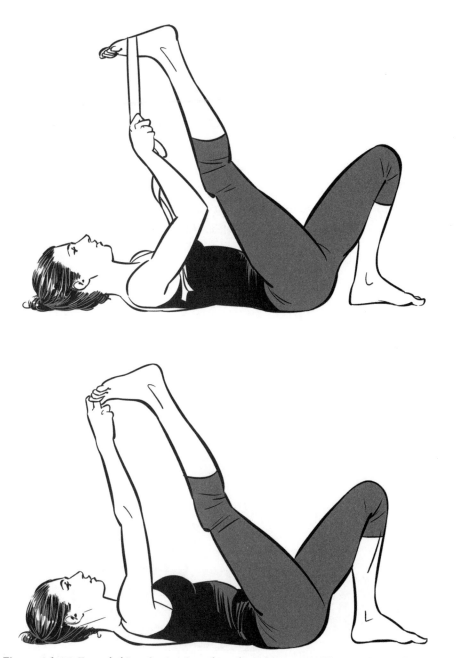

Figures 96–97, Extended Leg Supine Stretch to the Side Pose Modification (top to bottom)

Ananda Balasana (Happy Baby)

This may be my signature pose, the one that exemplifies Doron Yoga the best. I teach this in almost all my classes, not only for the stretching and releasing of spine and hips, but because we do this pose with a rolling laughter. I normally teach this pose after we do some intense backbends or core work—anytime we may begin to take ourselves too seriously, really. This reminds us of the joyful attitude we want to embody, a big reason of our practice—not just to get more flexible, but really enjoy life, and practice with ease. (**fig. 98**)

Method of practice: Lie down on your back, bend the knees, and bring the feet up, reaching for the feet with your hands, allowing the knees to drop towards the floor on either side of the body. Roll gently from side to side, massaging the spine and opening the hips. Feel free to allow a smile to come onto your face or even let your laughter roll out loud. This is great anytime, and especially when you want to release the back and hips, such as after a strong backbend.

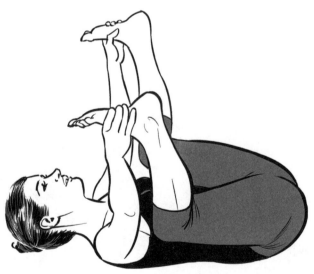

Figure 98, Happy Baby Pose

Malasana (Garland Pose/Squat)

A simple squatting pose that is practiced in India on a regular basis for washing clothes, waiting for the bus or going to the restroom. Apart from yoga practice, consider squatting every now and then, maybe as you enjoy some tea? (**fig. 99**)

Method of practice: From standing, begin to bend the knees and lower your hips back and down. Keep lowering down as far as you can. You may need to lift the heels up—that's fine. You may also need to externally rotate your feet. Over time you will be able to lower the heels down and keep the feet parallel.

Place the elbows to the inside of your knees and use the pressure of the elbows pressing against the knees to lengthen in the spine and open the heart.

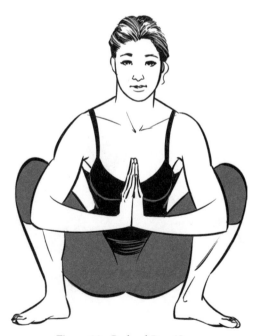

Figure 99, Garland Pose/Squat

Core Work

For all core work, make sure your belly is held in and does not puff out. While you are on your back, keep the lower back close to the ground so there is no arch. Arching the upper back is fine. Though I offer some dedicated core practices here, if you are using your bandhas, the core gets to work throughout the practice, especially when you jump through to sit, and jump back as well as in inversions and arm balances.

Basic Tips for Practicing Core Work

- Practice core work slowly and with awareness. Let it be just like any other yoga practice. Move with your breath. Exhale as you come up and inhale as you release.

- Stay calm throughout the core practice. Keep the mind and face relaxed.

- Practice to create stability and strength in the body, not for ego lifting. Set the intention to stay relaxed and enjoy the process.

**Navasana (Boat Pose)

Navasana (boat pose) is the classic core work of ashtanga vinyasa. It is a great pose, however it can create pressure on the lower back. All levels can practice this if modifying. Remember to breathe and keep a calm face. This is a great pose to practice stretching your lips to your ears. (Smile!) **(fig. 100)**

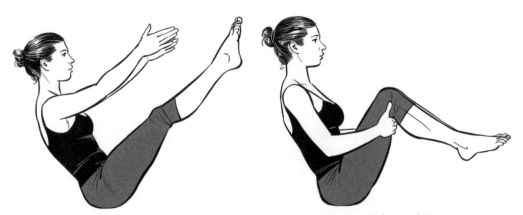

Figures 100–101, Boat Pose and Boat Pose Modification (left to right)

Method of practice: From a seated position, lift your legs up, straight if possible, to about face height. Lift your arms up, and have them straight toward the feet. Stay for five breaths and then release down. You can hug your legs in and straighten your spine, or you can practice crossing the legs and lifting your body up, hands on the floor, for a breath.

Traditionally this is repeated five times for five breaths each. I like doing three rounds, with the first round longer, about eight to ten breaths, and the second and third rounds for five breaths.

Modification: Keep the knees bent. This reduces the pressure from the back. If this is still too challenging, hold the back of the thighs with your hands. You can also start with hands in the air, and bring them to hold the thighs after you begin to fatigue. (**fig. 101, opposite page**)

**Bicycle Yoga*

Bicycle yoga is the ultimate core work that works all parts of the core—low abs, six-pack, and the side muscles of the core. Practice this as a meditation, slowly and with deep breaths. This can be practiced anytime. (**fig. 102**)

Method of practice: Lie down on your back. Bring your knees up to a 90-degree angle with the shins parallel to the floor. Clasp the hands behind the head and as you exhale, straighten the left leg forward keeping it about a foot off the floor.

At the same time, lift your torso, straighten the left arm and bring it to the outside of the right thigh. Then bring the right elbow towards the inner left elbow. Finish your exhale completely and as you inhale, lower the torso down, bend the left knee back beside the right knee, and adjust the arms into the original position.

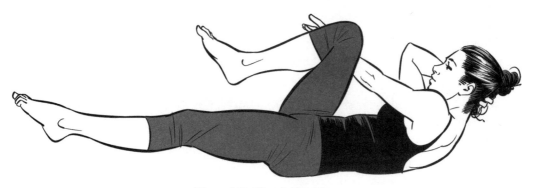

Figure 102, Bicycle Yoga Pose

Repeat on the right side and then continue on both sides, taking deep slow breaths. Make sure that you lift the torso up without compressing in the neck. You might not come as high up, but you will surely use your core. Repeat until you really feel the belly burning and then rest for a few breaths. You can repeat this once or twice more. This pose is wonderful as it works the upper, lower, and sides of the abs.

*Jatharasana (Leg Lifts)

The leg lifts are good core work practice, especially for the lower belly. Pay attention to lower back pain, and release if it hurts, or use your hands under the hips. (**fig. 103, opposite page**)

Method of practice: Lie down on your back placing the hands underneath your hips and lift your legs up to 90 degrees with your feet up towards the sky. With your exhale, slowly lower the legs down to a foot off the floor. Hold there while crisscrossing the legs for a count of five and then slowly lift the legs back up to 90 degrees while crisscrossing them. Repeat ten times or until you really feel the core working. This is most beneficial if you do it at least twice.

Modification: Skip the crisscrossing and if needed, lower one leg at a time and simply lift back up one leg at a time.

**Variation:* Lift the head and the upper shoulders off the ground and keep them lifted while doing the leg lifts. You may also want to try and place the hands at the heart or even overhead for maximum intensity. This will help to cultivate upper and lower belly strength.

*Core Leg Twists

Doing the core leg twists helps strengthen the side muscles of the core, which are many times overlooked. Practice slowly with deep breaths. (**fig. 104, opposite page**)

Method of practice: Lie down on your back and raise your legs up 90 degrees, feet towards the sky. Take your arms out to the sides in a "T" position with the palms facing down. As you exhale, lower the legs to the left until they are a foot off the floor. As you inhale, bring them back up, exhale, and lower them to a foot off the floor on the right side. As you inhale, bring them back up. Keep this going for as long as you can.

Modifications: Bend the knees as much as you need to so you can lower down close to the floor. Over time you can work on straightening the legs. You can start with fewer repetitions on each side and over time, increase the number of repetitions.

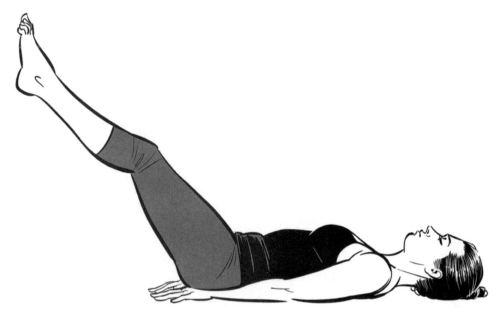

Figure 103, Leg Lift Pose

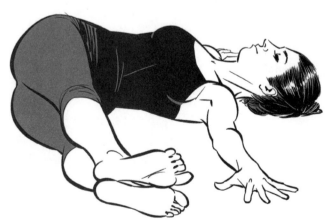

Figure 104, Core Leg Twist Pose

Arm Balances

Arm balances are great for toning the body, strengthening the core, arms, and shoulders, and improving our focus and balance. They are challenging for most and often involve some fear. They can be like a treat or playtime—an opportunity to practice with a smile and nonattachment. They can be humbling or ego inflators. Hopefully, you simply try to do them calmly and enjoy the process.

At times arm balances are called party poses, because some people get excited to see them while others enjoy showing them off. There have been some great teachers of the past that have used these poses to lure others into yoga—which is different than showing off for personal ego satisfaction. Work toward eventually practicing arm balances with grace and calm. They should become *stiram sukkah*—steady and with ease.

Basic Tips for Practicing Arm Balances

- Practice awareness of what happens in the body and mind before, during, and after the pose. Engage the bandhas.
- Shift the weight. Do not try to lift one side of the balancing body. Keep feeling a lift up rather than falling into gravity.
- Keep the arms engaged and push into the floor to engage the back and chest. The more stacked you are over the foundation (hands), especially in the hips, the easier it will be to balance.
- Keep the heart open as you practice and the gaze steadily down or slightly forward, not back.
- Play with pressing into the fingertips or the ball of the hands to move the body back into balance while you keep your weight distributed evenly on either side of your foundation (arms).
- Keep the legs active even when in the air.
- For the exit, lift the hips by taking the pubic bone further towards the tailbone. Once the pelvis tilts, the legs can follow. Keep bandhas engaged for landing.
- Keep breathing steadily. There is a tendency to hold the breath in arm balances. Practice staying steady and calm.

***Bakasana (Crow Pose)

Crow pose may be the most common arm balance in yoga. It strengthens the arms, the back, the core, and the chest, while demanding us to stay focused. (**fig. 105**)

Method of practice: Come to a squat position, lift your hips up, and place your knees onto your upper arms, as close to the armpits as possible. Bend the elbows and take your gaze forward so that you open the chest and relax the shoulders away from the ears. Begin shifting your weight forward so that the elbows come right over the wrists.

Keep the chest open and extending forward as you shift your weight of the hips to come over the arms. Your head will move forward, and the legs will come up slightly on their own.

Once you find balance, work on lifting your heels up higher towards your hips and straightening your arms. Keep your palms on the floor but allow your knuckles to come up slightly so, like a bird, you can move forward and back on the hands to help you with your balance.

Modification: It is best to learn this pose with a teacher present, but you may also want to place a blanket, or a sponge block, in front of you so that if you do fall forward, you have some padding.

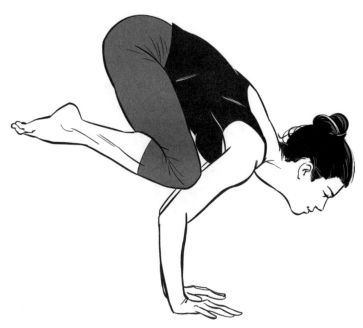

Figure 105, Crow Pose

Vasisthasana (Side Plank)

Side plank helps strengthen the core and shoulders. Great after you do other core work, or as a quick way to get some core work in when doing a shorter practice. (**fig. 106**)

Method of practice: Come into plank, turn your body sideways so that you're on your left hand and the left outer edge of your left foot. Stack the right foot on top of the left so that you are completely sideways. Take the right arm up the sky and lift the hips high. It can be a challenge to balance here, so activating your bandhas is key.

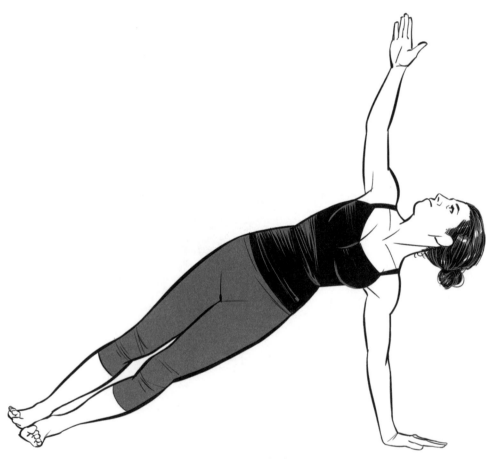

Figure 106, Side Plank Pose

Modification: Do the same pose with the bottom knee on the ground. Keep lifting the hips up while in the pose. (**fig. 107**)

For another modification that is just a bit more challenging: bend the top leg and place the foot flat on the ground either in front of or behind the other leg while continuing to lift the hips up. If you have any wrist discomfort, you can practice the same pose on your forearm.

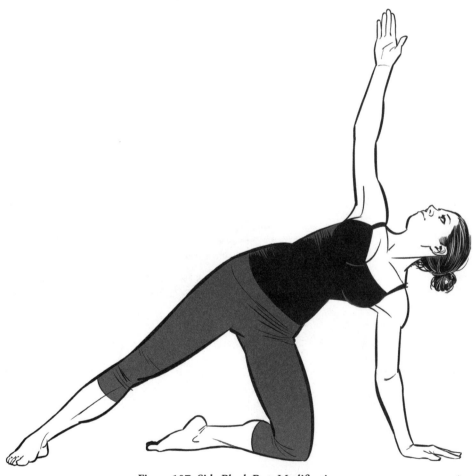

Figure 107, Side Plank Pose Modification

***Variations:* Lift the top leg while in side plank. You can hold it here in the air for a few breaths. If available, place the leg that is in the air in a tree pose, or you can try to hold your toe with the peace sign fingers, which will stretch your hamstrings as well and challenge your balance. Take your gaze to the sky, and keep your tailbone tucked under. (**fig. 108**)

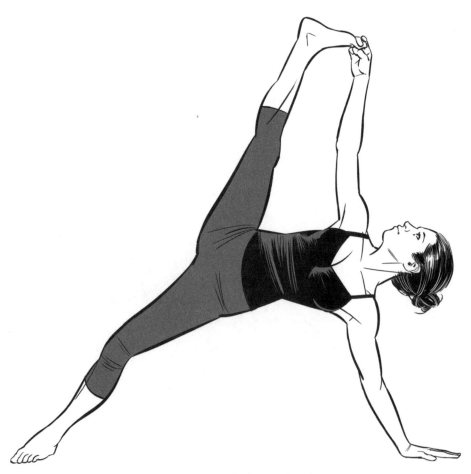

Figure 108, Side Plank Pose Variation

Backbends/Back Extensions

Backbends, as they are commonly known, do bend the back but also help extend the back and create more space between the vertebrae and overall length in the spine.

Backbends also stretch the entire front of the body, thus they are sometimes called heart openers. They are great for balancing the modern lifestyle habits that require us to lean or bend forward. As heart openers, they also help expand the chest area and the emotional heart center, which allows for more openness and ability to truly feel and experience life in general and relationships in particular.

Backbends are stimulating, energizing, and warming.

Basic Tips for Practicing Backbends

- Take a moment to relax your mind before moving into a backbend.
- Begin with activation of mulabandha (root control center). Lengthen the belly and mid back and keep lengthening up to the thoracic spine (upper back) so that the curve spreads throughout the spine.
- Lift and expand your heart center for physical and emotional opening.
- Move the sacrum in and up towards the navel and roll the thighs inward.
- Keep the shoulders relaxed to protect the neck. Shoulders should rotate externally, keeping space between the shoulder blades.
- Maintain your ujjayi breath (victorious breath). There is a tendency to hold the breath in intense backbends. Use your inhales for lifting in the chest area and exhales to keep calm.
- Take the knees from side to side to release between sets of backbends, and do a twist followed by forward folds at the end. Listen to your body, and do not go beyond what feels safe. Patience is a virtue.

Shalabhasana (Locust)

Locust strengthens the back of the body. Great for preventing back pain, though if you already have back pain, do not push into it, but rather practice gently. **(fig. 109)**

Method of practice: Lie down on your belly and place the hands alongside the body, palms facing up. Keeping the feet close together, lift the chest and the legs. Keep the spine long and tuck the tailbone under. Keep the head reaching forward so the neck stays long. Breathe deeply for five to eight breaths.

*Variation: As you lift up, clasp the hands behind the back and use that leverage to lift a little higher by reaching the arms away from the body. **(fig. 110)**

Modification: If you feel too much pressure on the hipbones or the groin, you may place a blanket underneath your hips.

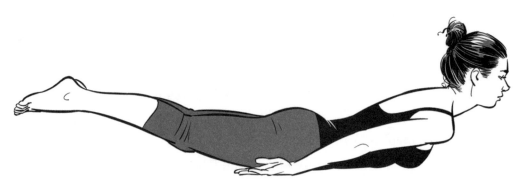

Figure 109, Locust Pose

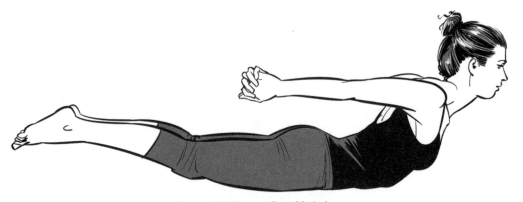

Figure 110, Locust Pose Variation

Setu Bandha Sarvangasana (Bridge)

Bridge is the classic preparation for upward bow. It is safe for all, and can be repeated a few times. As in all backbends, if there is back pain, do not push through it, but rather focus on lengthening more than deepening. (**fig. 111**)

Method of practice: Lie down on your back. Bring the knees up, placing the feet on the floor, parallel to each other. Now tuck the tailbone towards the feet (creating space for L4–L5), then lift the hips, clasp the hands underneath the back, and roll your shoulders in so that you create space for the neck. Keep lifting the hips, moving the chest towards the chin and the chin slightly back away from the chest.

Hold for five deep breaths and release. Allow your knees to drop from one side to the other a couple of times and repeat two more times.

Modification: Take your feet further away from your hips. The closer your feet are to your hips, the more intense your pose will be, so adjust as necessary. You can also place a block underneath your lower back for a more relaxed variation.

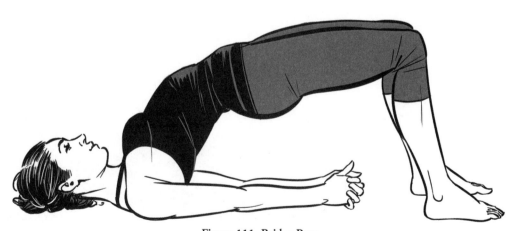

Figure 111, Bridge Pose

Ardha Bhekasana (Half Frog/Quad Stretch)

Half frog is a great quad stretch and a gentle backbend. It can become a deeper backbend when you lift higher, so move slowly. Do not push through knee pain. If it hurts in the knee, stop and check with a professional on how to do it right. You can also visit the Doronyoga channel on YouTube for many pose explanations. **(fig. 112)**

Method of practice: Lie down on your belly. Place the left forearm parallel to the front of the mat, bend the right knee, and with your right hand, slowly bring the knee forward towards the floor.

Consider rotating in the shoulder and taking the right elbow up to sky while rotating the wrist in order to bring the fingers forward in the same direction as the toes, just like chaturanga (low push up) arms.

Keep the right foot parallel to the body while bringing it alongside the body. Don't let the foot twist sideways. Press your body up to get a slight backbend as well.

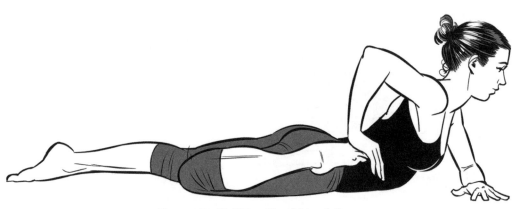

Figure 112, Half Frog/Quad Stretch Pose

Salamba Bhujangasana (Sphinx/Supported Cobra)

Sphinx is the best foundation pose for understanding backbends. It is safe and a good place to work on the basics. I use the feeling I have in my chest doing sphinx, while practicing many other poses such as arm balances and some inversions. (**fig. 113**)

Method of practice: Lie down on your belly and then come up to your forearms. Keep the shoulders over the elbows and the elbows in. Root your hands into the earth and lightly pull forward so that you can feel more space in the lower back. Feel how you are moving forward first and then up, creating a back extension. Keep the feet parallel and rooting into the ground.

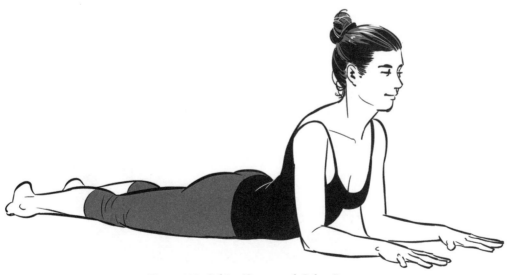

Figure 113, Sphinx/Supported Cobra Pose

Bhujangasana (Cobra)

Cobra is a yoga classic, and a great way to open the chest and stretch the spine, and can substitute upward facing dog anytime. Don't forget to breathe! (**fig. 114**)

Method of practice: Lie down on your belly. Place your hands under your shoulders and lift the chest forward and up. Keep the elbows slightly bent no matter how much you have opened your chest.

Make sure to keep lengthening the lower back as you open your chest by moving both the chest forward and the tailbone down and back.

Keep the knees and feet on the ground. Lengthen the neck without over-extending backward. Keep pressing all ten fingers into the ground.

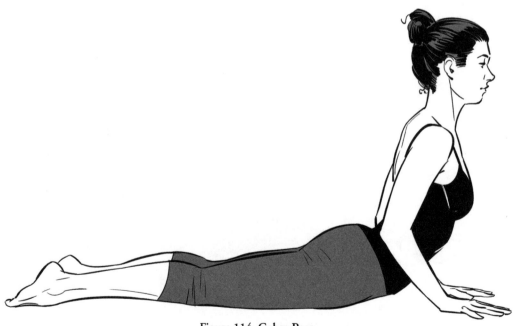

Figure 114, Cobra Pose

Modification: If your back is sensitive, lift just to the point where you can lift the hands off the floor and stay up. (**fig. 115**)

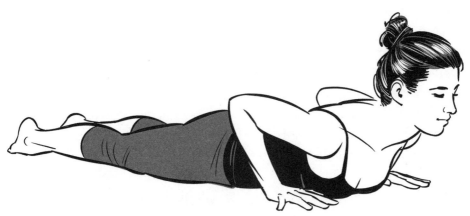

Figure 115, Cobra Pose Modification

**Dhanurasana (Bow Pose)

Bow pose is a backbend that helps prepare for upward bow. You can practice this once or up to three times with a few breaths break between each round. Remember to breath in the pose. (**fig. 116, opposite page**)

Method of practice: Lie down on the belly, bend the knees, and reach your hands back to hold the ankles. Press the legs back and up and lift the chest off the ground. Lift the chest forward and up to create extension as you open up. Bring the feet to touch and the knees hip-width apart.

Modification: If it is hard to reach the ankles, you can hold the feet. If this hurts the groin, you can place a blanket underneath the hips.

***Variation:* As this pose gets easier, hold the legs farther down the ankles or shins.

**Ustrasana (Camel Pose)

Camel pose is a backbend that works with gravity. This means that your work is simply to slow down the bending and make sure it does not happen too deep too fast. (**fig. 117, opposite page**)

Method of practice: The classic pose is done by placing your knees on your mat. I like to use a blanket or fold my mat for extra knee padding. Begin by placing your hands on your hips. With an inhalation, lengthen your spine up, and as you exhale begin arching back towards the feet. Move your hands back onto your ankles. Keep lifting your chest up with every inhalation, as well as move your hips forward. Try and keep the hips over the knees as much as you can.

To exit the pose, press the hips forward, and vertabrae by vertabrae, lift up. Let the head be the last to lift up. This may seem counter intuitive, but when you lift the head first, you actually create a collapse in the chest that blocks you from lifting up, and can be dangerous for the back. So remember, for safety: head last. Also, when coming up, try and come up evenly with the spine, so that you are not lifting one side first—again, for the safety of your back. Take child's pose or a vinyasa, and repeat.

Modification: If reaching back to the heels is too far, you can begin by keeping the hands on the hips and simply bend back as far as it feels okay on your back. When this is comfortable, tuck your toes under and reach for the heels. This way, the heels are a bit higher—thus closer to your hands.

Most important is to remember to breathe while in the pose, as well as in your transition in and out of it.

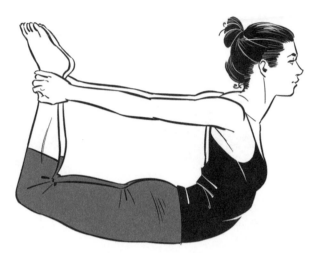

Figure 116, Bow Pose

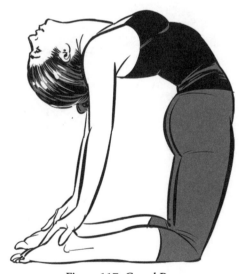

Figure 117, Camel Pose

***Urdhva Dhanurasana (Upward Facing Bow)*

Welcome to the ultimate backbend. This pose requires open shoulders, back, and hip flexors. Try to notice where you feel most limited and stretch that area separately before doing this pose. Most Doron Yoga sequences make sure you warm up all these body parts before you practice the upward facing bow. You can always stay with bridge pose as a substitute. (**figs. 118–119**)

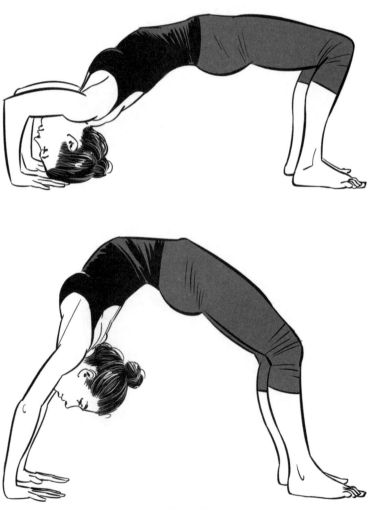

Figures 118–119, Upward Facing Bow Pose (top to bottom)

Method of practice: Lie down on your back. Bring the knees up, placing the feet on the floor parallel to each other. Place your hands next to the ears, lift the hips up, and press up to your head. Adjust the elbows so that they are parallel to one another, and move them over the wrists; then press up to straighten the arms. Make sure not to press straight up, but rather feel the lower back extend towards the knees as the chest moves towards the hands. Keep the feet parallel to each other and the knees moving toward each other. This will help protect the back. Over time, walk the hands towards the feet, while maintaining an arch in the spine.

Note: It is better not to do this pose until you can do it with almost straight arms.

Modification: Lift only to your head. Stay for a few breaths and release. When doing so, try keeping the elbows parallel to each other. If your shoulders are tight it will require some work squeezing the elbows in towards each other. You can rotate your hands slightly outward to help with the elbow movement. This helps keep space between the shoulder blades and protects your neck and shoulders from stress.

*Variation: This variation can be either a preparation for the upward facing bow, or actually take you deeper and prepare you for the full drop back (lowering to the backbend from standing position). (**fig. 120, next page**)

Method of practice: As a preparation for the upward facing bow, stand with your back facing a wall and take the arms over the head towards the wall. Walk the hands down the wall as far as you can without bending the knees or going into your backbend yet.

Keep the elbows parallel and try to lift the chest to the sky while pressing the hips forward (away from the wall). Breathe deeply. This will help open the shoulders and the back.

If upward facing bow is very comfortable, you can try and work on going deeper, preferably with the guidance of a qualified teacher. To prepare for the drop backs, you will continue to walk the hands down the wall, just to the place you feel comfortable. (Remember you still need to come back up!) Stay for five calm breaths, and walk back up.

The exit is the same as in ustrasana (camel pose)—vertebrae by vertebrae with the head lifting last. Always practice three upward facing bow poses, before you go to the wall, to ensure you are sufficiently warmed up. I like to simply forward fold standing for a few breaths before I continue with the twists and seated forward folds. Do what feels good in your body.

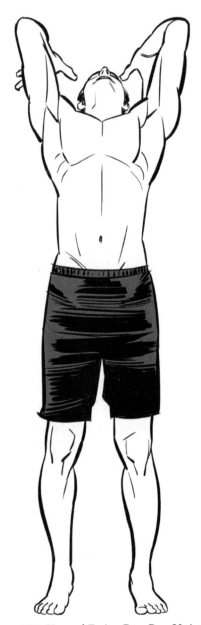

Figure 120, Upward Facing Bow Pose Variation

***Eka Pada Raj Kapotasana (One Legged King Pigeon Pose)

One legged king pigeon pose is a deep backbend that stretches the entire front of the body as well as the back. It requires open shoulders, hips, hip flexors, and of course back. Be patient with this pose. It took me over a decade to do it fully. Every step of the process is an opening, on the physical level, emotional level, and even spiritual. As you open your heart and back here, you may feel some release of emotional blockages and a clearer flow of energy through the body. (**fig. 121**)

Method of practice: From *adho mukha svanasana* (downward facing dog), bring your left foot forward, so that the left knee goes behind and a bit to the outside of the left wrist. The left foot will go out as far as is comfortable for your hips and knee. Lower your hips down, reach back and take your right foot with your hands over the head. This is a deep backbend that stretches the front of the thigh, back, and shoulders. Be very careful with this pose and go slowly.

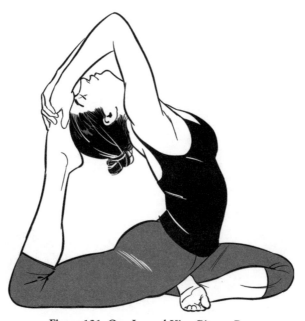

Figure 121, One Legged King Pigeon Pose

Modification: See eka pada raj kapotasana prep (pigeon pose), for some great ways to open the hips and prepare for this pose. I practice the prep regularly as it really helps open the hips.

Variation:* If you are comfortable with the prep version, you may want to reach one hand behind and work on bringing the back foot forward. (figs. 122–123**)

If this is comfortable, try lifting your left arm up in the air so that you start to stretch your shoulder and learn to balance without hand support.

Then, if you are comfortable, shift the hand holding the leg so that the foot is in the elbow crease. Then try to take the other hand over the head and clasp the hands behind you.

You can also do this with a strap between the hands. Make sure you keep lifting the upper chest to protect your lower back. Work on squaring the chest forward.

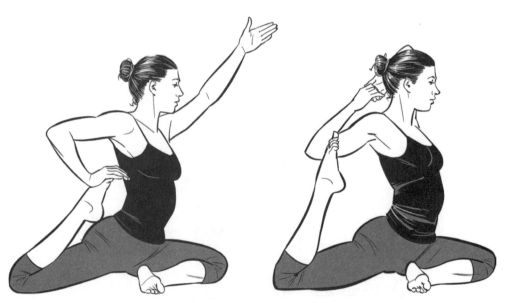

Figures 122–123, One Legged King Pigeon Pose Variation (left to right)

Inversions

Inversions are fun and rewarding. They help us overcome fear, create strength and stability, and become okay with being upside down. Inversions help focus and steady the mind.

Inversions can be slightly intimidating at first and are best learned with a teacher present. You can use the wall when you first learn these poses. Practice against the wall until you feel steady and ready to move towards the center of the room.

Lying down with the legs up the wall is the most basic form of inversions, and for some this will be enough. Once inversions are mastered, they can be grounding, calming, and healing.

Basic Tips for Practicing Inversions

- Activate the bandhas, and keep them active during transitions as well as while in the pose. Keep the shoulders away from the ears and maintain space between the shoulder blades.

- Shift the weight of the hips over the shoulders, to help transition into the inversion. Keep the legs active even when they are in the air.

- Keep the gaze steady and the mind focused, and keep your breath alive and smooth.

- Press your support (head, hands, elbows) into the ground to help you lift.

- Stay calm and try to relax into the pose. Be attentive to your body. Headstands (*sirsasana*) and shoulder stands (*salamba sarvangasana*) can pose risks to the neck and should always be practiced with care.

Viparita Karani (Inverted Action, Legs up the Wall)

Legs up the wall can be practiced by anyone, anytime. No need for warm up, and it is safe even for women on their cycle. It can substitute any other inversion offered in the Doron Yoga sequences, and can also be practiced anytime you need to restore. When teaching a few classes a day, I would sometimes take this pose for five minutes between classes to restore my energy and stay grounded. It is safe to stay here even longer, and practice leg variations (reclined wide legs and reclined bound angle) as well. (**fig. 124**)

Method of practice: Sitting sideways next to a wall, bring your left hip as close to the wall as possible, then lift the legs up towards the wall as you twist to bring both hips to face the wall.

The legs should be straight up the wall while the arms rest alongside the body, or place your left hand on the belly and your right hand on the chest and focus on your breath flowing through your belly and chest. To come out of the pose, bend the knees and roll onto one side. You may want to use a blanket underneath your hips for comfort.

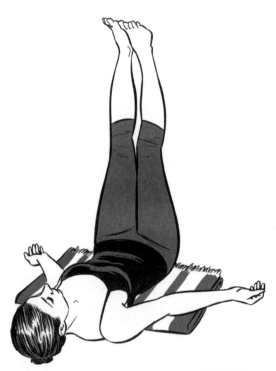

Figure 124, Inverted Action, Legs up the Wall Pose

Supta Upavishta Konasana (Reclined Wide Legs)

I used the reclined wide legs pose in order to open quicker into *upavishta konasana* (seated wide leg stretch). The beauty of this pose is that you can be in it for fifteen minutes and simply relax. I like taking deep breaths here and allowing my body and mind to simply surrender. You will notice how much you actually did when you exit the pose, so release slowly and with care. (**fig. 125**)

Method of practice: From legs straight up the wall, begin to open them slowly as wide as feels comfortable for you while still resting on the wall. Stay in the pose for three to fifteen minutes. Make sure to come out very slowly and with the support of the hands.

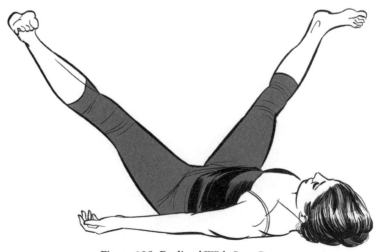

Figure 125, Reclined Wide Legs Pose

Supta Baddha Konasana (Reclined Bound Angle)

Reclined bound angle is very relaxing and can be held for long durations. You can even begin your *savasana* (corpse—final relaxation) this way. For some people, this may feel better on the back than having the legs straight. It will help open the hips in a gentle way. (**fig. 126**)

Method of practice: Lie down on your back. Bring the feet together and open your knees to the side. Let your knees fall towards the floor. Allow your body to relax as much as possible. Stay here for as long as it feels good.

Modification: For a more restorative variation, place support such as blocks or blankets under the knees.

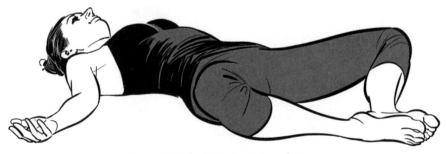

Figure 126, Reclined Bound Angle Pose

Variation: From viparita karani (legs up the wall), bring the soles of your feet together and your knees apart. Lower the knees down towards your hips, and let your body relax into the pose. Stay for as long as it feels good. (**fig. 127**)

In all of the legs up the wall poses, really allow your body to relax. You can place a blanket or a bolster underneath your hips to support your back.

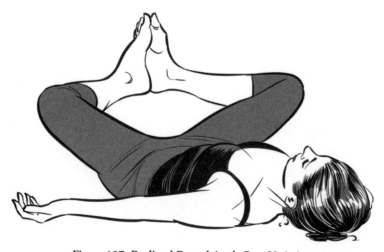

Figure 127, Reclined Bound Angle Pose Variation

Salamba Sarvangasana (Shoulder Stand)

Some call the shoulder stand the queen of poses, as it is said to be very healing on many levels, including balancing hormones and a variety of illnesses. Whether true or not, this pose is practiced by almost all yoga styles and as long as it feels okay on your neck, it is a safe way to invert, reverse the flow of blood, move energy, calm, and stabilize. Try to practice it as a meditation, staying in stillness for some time (from ten breaths to five minutes). (**fig. 128**)

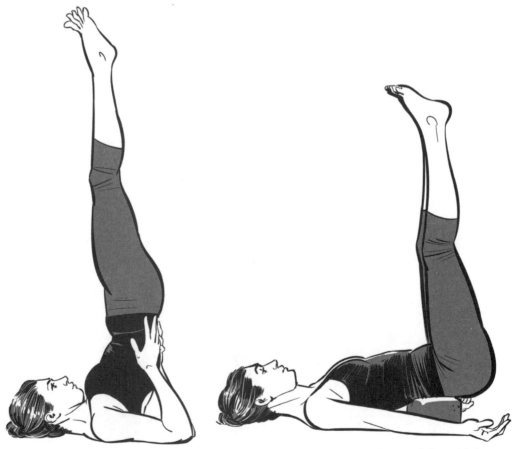

Figures 128–129, Shoulder Stand Pose and Shoulder Stand Pose Modification (left to right)

Method of practice: Lie down on your back. Lift your legs and take them over the head. Place your hands on your back and roll your shoulders underneath to create more space for your neck. Try to keep your elbows parallel to each other.

Extend the legs up towards the sky and take your gaze to your feet or watch your breath rise and fall at your belly. Keep lifting from your feet up, and if possible, walk the hands up the back (closer to the floor).

If there is pressure on the neck, you may need to place a blanket underneath the shoulders and have your head on the mat or floor. This elevates the shoulders and creates space for the neck. You can also try moving the chin away from the chest to create some more space for the neck. It is best to get advice from a teacher. Once up, stay calm and focused, and try to breathe deeply.

Modification: Place a block underneath the lower back and raise the legs straight up. This way you can be in a more relaxed state but still get the benefits of inverting. This is very useful for days when energy is low or for women who are menstruating. (**fig. 129, opposite page**)

Halasana (Plow Pose)

Plow pose is a deep forward fold (upside down), so move gently especially if you have back pain. You can always bend the knees, either just a bit, or go directly into ear pressure pose. (fig. 130)

Method of practice: From salamba sarvangasana (shoulder stand), lower the legs straight over the head. If they reach the ground, untuck your toes. Stay for five to ten breaths.

Modification: This may not be possible, or may be too intense on the back. If so, bend the knees just enough to allow you to lower the legs. Try and keep them somewhat straight even if you are not lowering very far down.

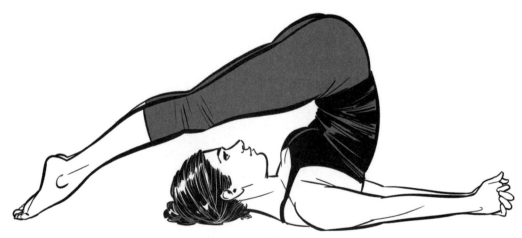

Figure 130, Plow Pose

Karnapidasana (Ear Pressure Pose)

Ear pressure pose is a bit safer for the spine than plow pose as the knees are bent. However still pay attention to your spine. (**fig. 131**)

Method of practice: From halasana (plow pose), bend the knees towards the ears. Stay here for five to ten breathes. To come out of karnapidasana (ear pressure pose), place your hands on the mat and use them to slow down your descent. Use your core muscles while lowering down.

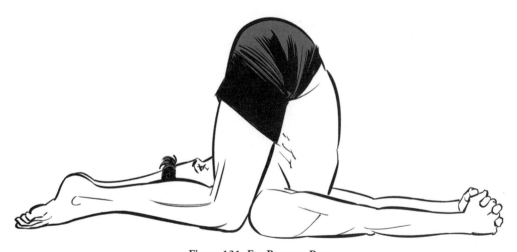

Figure 131, Ear Pressure Pose

Matsyasana (Fish Pose)

Matsyasana (fish pose) is a counter pose for the shoulder stand. It stretches the neck and throat in the opposite direction of the shoulder stand. (**fig. 132, opposite page**)

Method of practice: Prop up onto your elbows, lift the chest, and allow the head to drop back towards the floor. If your head does not reach the floor, move your elbows towards the feet, until you can reach your head to the ground. Stay for ten breaths while lifting the chest up.

Modification: If this is uncomfortable on your lower back, place your hands under your hips. This will ease the backbend.

*Vayu Muktyasana (Knees to the Chest Pose)

Knees to the chest is a nice gentle forward fold (on the back). Though this pose can be done anytime, it is a great counter pose to the fish pose. (**fig. 133, opposite page**)

Method of practice: When you are done with fish, simply bring your knees to the chest for a few breaths. You can even roll gently from side to side on your back while doing this. It is a feel-good pose.

**Shoulder Stand Sequence

Shoulder stand is always done as sequence of poses. (**fig. 134, opposite page**)

Method of practice: First come up to shoulder stand, and stay there for ten breaths. Then lower the legs down over the head into halasana (plow pose) for eight breaths followed by bending the knees toward the ears into karnapidasana (ear pressure pose) for eight breaths. Place your hands on the mat, and lower your legs slowly down. Prop onto your elbows to take matsyasana (fish pose) for eight breaths and finish with knees to the chest for five breaths.

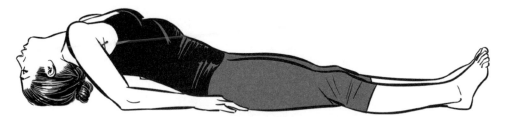

Figure 132, Fish Pose

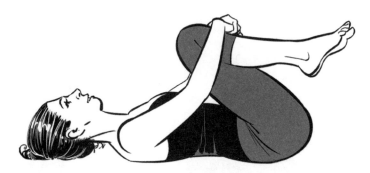

Figure 133, Knees to the Chest Pose

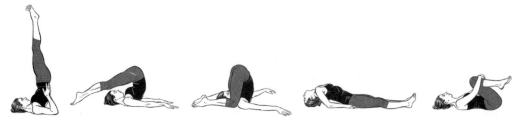

Figure 134, Shoulder Stand Sequence Pose *(left to right:
salamba sarvangasana, halasana, karnapidasana, matsyasana, vayu muktyasana)*

***Sirsasana (Headstand)

Headstand is practiced for grounding, inverting, gaining balance, and focus, and some yogis in India claim that this pose has many other health benefits. At times it is called king of poses. Avoid it if you have neck pain, and be careful if you have back pain (especially in the transitions), though it may actually be helpful to have the spine hanging upside down (consider an inversion therapy that does not have pressure on the head for releasing the back). (**figs. 135–138, pages 196–197**)

Method of practice: Come to all fours and then lower down to your elbows. Hold opposite elbows with the hands. Keeping your elbows where they are, open up your hands and clasp them together, placing the outer edges of your hands on the mat.

Place the crown of the head onto the floor so that the back of the head is pressing against the hands. Press the elbows down and lift the shoulders up and away from your ears. Tuck the toes under and lift the knees, coming into downward dog with headstand variation. Walk the feet towards the head as far as you can. You will need to lift in the belly and extend the hips tall to keep from rolling over.

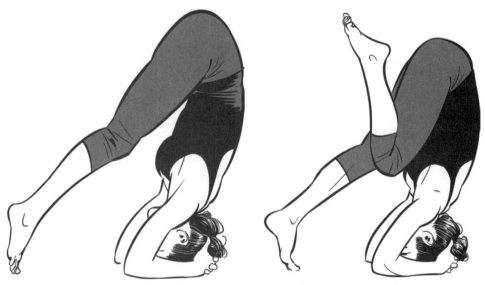

Figures 135–136, Headstand Pose (left to right) (cont. next page)

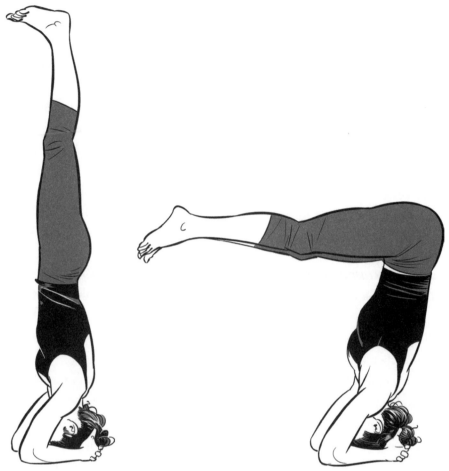

(cont.) Figures 137–138, Headstand Pose (left to right)

Lift your right leg up keeping the knee bent and press strongly into the elbows. Lift in the belly and if available, raise the left leg with the knee bent so that now your hips are over the shoulders and your legs are in the air with the knees bent. When you feel steady, press the legs up, reaching the balls of the feet towards the sky and squeeze the ankles together while maintaining the lift in the belly. The more you are stacked in one vertical line, the easier it will be.

To come down, slowly begin lowering the legs with knees bent or straight, balancing the weight of the legs by slightly moving the hips back. Not much movement is needed in the hips, just enough to counter the weight of the legs as you come down. Most of the work will be done in the core. Once down, take balasana (child's pose) to rest for a few breaths.

If you roll over while straightening up to the sky, simply release the clasp of the hands and allow yourself to roll. Smile and try again. Make sure to take child's pose when you are finished with your headstand.

Modification: While in the downward dog headstand, lift one leg up and hold it for ten breaths. Lower down, and then do the other side.

****Variation:* While in headstand, lower the legs halfway down and then bring them back up. Move slowly and repeat three to five times. If you still have energy, come down halfway once more and hold. Save a bit of energy to come back up and then lower all the way to the floor.

Sirsasana can be practiced with many variations, including padmasana (lotus), upavishta konasana (bound angle), and more. Once you are steady and know how to balance your weight, you are welcome to play around.

****Pincha Mayurasana (Dolphin Pose to Forearm Balance/Feathered Peacock)*

Forearm balance is a good pose for strengthening the back and shoulders. Like other inversions, it helps build confidence, stability, focus, and a sense of power. Start practicing against the wall until you feel safe and steady to do this in the middle of the room—preferably with a teacher. **(figs. 139–140, opposite page)**

Method of practice: Come to all fours and then lower down to the forearms so that the elbows are underneath the shoulders and the hands are in line with the shoulders. Press your thumbs and index fingers firmly into the mat. Press your elbows down, and lift your shoulders up and away from the ears while tucking your toes under and lifting your hips to the sky.

Bring your gaze forward to the hands and walk your feet forward towards the head as far as you can, making sure your shoulders stay over the elbows and you are maintaining the lift in the belly and the upward lengthen in the torso to keep from rolling over. This is the dolphin pose—the preparation pose for the full forearm balance.

Take your right leg up to the sky, keeping it as straight as possible. Bend the left knee and kick the left foot up to meet the right, making sure you straighten and activate the left leg as you are coming up so you are consciously using effort to lift the left leg to meet the right. Use the lift in the belly to help you come up and to keep you steady.

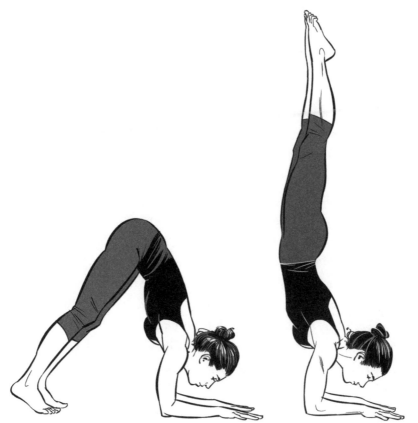

Figures 139–140, Dolphin Pose to Forearm Balance/Feathered Peacock Pose (left to right)

Keep pressing your elbows down and lifting the shoulders up, as that will activate the muscles of your upper back, especially your latissimus dorsi. The lattisimus dorsi are sometimes called lats. They are broad muscles on the back that help support your balance—somewhat like wings—so keep them active!

Modification: Stay in dolphin (forearm downward dog), and practice pressing the elbows firmly into the ground so that you activate the chest, shoulders, and back muscles. When this gets easy, you can do the same thing with one leg lifted straight up to the sky and hold for ten deep breaths. If this is all too much, do your dolphin with the knees on the ground. This will help build the strength in the shoulders and upper body. Try to hold it until you really feel the shoulders burn.

Adho Mukha Vrksasana (Handstand)

Although handstands are practiced in gymnastics, recently they have carved their space in the yoga world. Remember that practicing handstands is fun, but not a requirement for yoga. Practice with a smile, use the wall, and above all enjoy and be happy with where you are. (**fig. 141, opposite page**)

Method of practice: Place your hands about shoulder-width apart on the ground. Move your weight forward over the wrists and lengthen the spine. With one leg at a time or both legs together, lift up to a handstand.

When coming up, focus on getting the hips over the shoulders first, and then follow with your legs. If you are kicking one leg at a time, take one leg straight up into the air. Bend the other one for the kick up, and straighten it as soon as it is in the air, while actively reaching it towards the sky. Once your legs are both up, squeeze the feet together; keep your belly lifted, your tailbone tucked under, and your gaze steady between the thumbs. Remember to breathe.

**Variations:* Handstand is a challenging pose and there are a few ways to prepare for it. The first one is to practice the L shape (see below), and once you get strong enough doing the L shape, you can begin practicing the full handstand with the wall. Eventually—probably with the help of a teacher—you will start to practice with no wall, but even if you never do, it is absolutely fine. Practicing with the wall will give you all the strengthening you need.

**L Shape

Sit on the ground facing the wall with your legs extended forward. Place your hand along the hips or even a few inches behind the hips. This is where you want the hands to be. Now turn around, placing the hands at the spot you "measured" and start climbing your legs up the wall behind you. The beginning position looks like a downward dog pose with the feet near the wall.

From there simply take one leg up to the wall, and then the other. You can stay in the L shape or work on lifting one leg up towards the sky while the other still presses against the wall. It is actually easier to hold with one leg up toward the sky. Switch legs. If you need to, come down between sides. Over time, try to increase the amount of time you hold each side. This will help build the strength and stamina you will need for the full handstand.

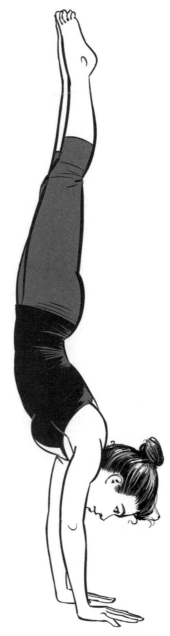

Figure 141, Handstand Pose

**Handstand Against the Wall

Come to downward dog position with your hands about a foot away from the wall. Walk the feet forward so that the shoulders are over the wrists and your gaze is between your thumbs. Bend your knees, lift in the belly, and hop, taking the hips over the shoulders and the legs up to the sky or the heels against the wall. At first, practice hopping with one leg at a time, and once that becomes easy, try hopping with both legs together.

Remember that the work is to get the hips over the shoulders and then the legs follow. Once up, try to adjust your lower back so that you are lifting in the belly and tucking the tailbone towards your feet. Stay here or practice moving away from the wall one leg at a time.

***Sirsasana B (Tripod Headstand)

There are many headstand variations, but the two I offer in this book are the most common. For some this pose is more accessible than sirsasana A (headstand A). You can always switch between the two. (**fig. 142, opposite page**)

Method of practice: Come to all fours, then lower the head to the floor and walk the hands back so that you create a 90-degree angle with bent elbows, which means that your upper arms will be parallel to the mat. Keep your shoulders in and over the wrists. Lifting in the belly, press strongly into the hands, activating the shoulders and moving them up and away from the ears.

Tuck the toes under, lift the knees, and take the hips up towards the sky. Walk the feet forward towards the arms while lifting in the belly and lengthening the spine towards the sky. Lift both legs up to the sky, or lift one at a time if necessary, stacking ankles over hips and hips over shoulders.

To come down, slowly begin lowering the legs with knees bent or straight, balancing the weight of the legs by slightly moving the hips back. Not much movement is needed in the hips, just enough to counter the weight of the legs as you come down. Most of the work will be done in the core. You can take child's pose to rest after this pose.

Modification: From the downward facing dog in tripod position, take your right knee onto your right upper arm as close to the armpit as possible. Either stay and breathe here, or bring the left knee onto the left upper arm. Once you have both legs up, stay for a few breaths or possibly work your way towards lifting into the full tripod headstand.

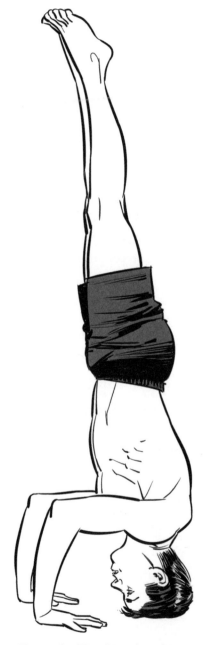

Figure 142, Tripod Headstand Pose

Even if you just have one leg up on the upper arm while the head is down, you are still practicing an inversion and getting its benefits. Take your time and slowly go through the options until you manage to make your way all the way upside down. Remember to practice no judgment.

***Variation:* When coming back down, slowly bend the knees, keeping the hips over the shoulders and lowering the knees towards the upper arms, keeping the hips over the shoulders for as long as you can. Eventually the hips will drop some, but by then you will be almost at arm level, and it will be easier to lower down. Stay for three to five breaths and either lift back up, drop back into chaturanga, or simply lower the feet down and come out of the pose. Take child's pose.

Finishing Poses

When you are done with the active part of your practice, it is important to integrate all you have done. The classic pose that should not be skipped is *savasana* (corpse pose). To that you may add a seated meditation before or after *savasana*. You can also practice some *pranayama*, thus integrating the other two parts of the Yoga Lifestyle into the yoga asana.

Tips for Practicing Finishing Poses

- Surrender. The active practice is over. Allow yourself to be whole. No need to work any specific part of the body.
- Enjoy! This is the treat at the end of your practice.

Savasana (Corpse/Final Relaxation)

Savasana (the final relaxation) is maybe the most important pose of them all. It is where we integrate all that we practiced so far, and allow the body to relax completely, with no control of our mind over it. It is called corpse pose because our practice is to let all control go, and be like a corpse—doing absolutely nothing. Not to be missed! (**fig. 143, opposite page**)

Method of practice: Lie down on your back and allow your feet to splay out to the sides. Let your arms rest to the sides of your body with the palms facing up.

Lift your chin slightly to the chest and rest your head down so your neck is long. Take a couple of big inhales, and with your exhales, feel your body surrender heavily into the floor while finding lightness in your mind. In this pose, we focus on nothing, allowing the body to just rest on its own and allowing the mind to stay calm and still. It is a complete relaxation pose.

Since it is not easy for many of us to find complete stillness or even total relaxation in the body, it may be helpful to scan the entire body. Start with the feet, allowing them to relax while keeping your awareness on them as they soften. Keep going up the body—to your calves, knees, thighs, hips, chest, shoulders, arms, hands, and finally, head. Take your time and really notice how every part that you focus on finds a bit more ease and surrender. We have a tendency to hold on to even little muscles without noticing. When you reach the head, scan all parts of your face from the forehead to the eyes, nose, jaw, and chin. Then finish with a calming of the mind by allowing your awareness to drop back into your breath.

Modification: If you feel any tension in the lower back, consider placing a bolster or rolled blanket under the backs of your knees.

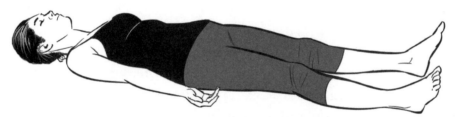

Figure 143, Corpse/Final Relaxation Pose

Yoga Sequences

Now that you have seen many yoga poses and even learned how to do them, it is time to put them together. Creating a sequence for a practice is an art. No worries; you will be given complete practices with images, but some things repeat themselves and it would be good to define them first. In all sequences, you will be prompted at times to "take a vinyasa," and many sequences start with the warm-up 1 and 2 and then follow with surya A, B (sun salutes A, B) and their variations, so first, here is a description of what these mean.

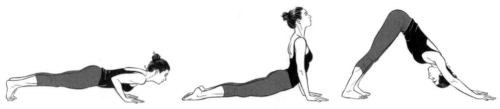

Figure 144, Vinyasa Sequence (left to right)

*Vinyasa

When we speak of vinyasa traditionally, we speak of a sequence that includes movement and breath placed in a certain way. For example, raising the arms overhead with an inhalation is the first vinyasa of the sun salutation. For our purposes of creating practice sequences, we will use the term vinyasa to describe a specific sequence of a few poses that we repeat often. There are different starting points from which you will arrive at chaturanga (low push up): maybe plank, maybe jumping back from ardha uttanasana (forward fold half way), or maybe lowering from warrior 1. (**fig. 144**)

THE VINYASA SEQUENCE

Use the vinyasa to keep the body warm and balance forward folds with backbends. Your first vinyasa may already be in the warm up 1 sequence. Maybe you will skip it here, or modify with knees down in chaturanga and a gentler backbend than upward dog, such as baby cobra. Keep doing vinyasas between your sun salutes to really warm up. During your practice you can use these to balance your dosha (body type). If you feel vata (air, distracted), do them slowly, if you feel vet pitta (fire, aggressive), skip some, and if you feel kapha (earth, lethargic), please add them between all seated poses.

- Exhale; lower to low plank (chaturanga dandasana).
- Inhale; move forward and up to upward facing dog (urdhva mukha svanasana).
- Exhale; roll over your toes, moving your hips back and up into downward facing dog (adho mukha svanasana).

Modification 1: From plank pose, lower the knees, the chest, and the chin, and then slide forward into a baby cobra or sphinx pose. Plant the hands on the floor, and starting with the knees down, lift your hips up and back, returning to downward facing dog.

Modification 2: If you are comfortable with lowering the knees, chest, and chin to the ground, try to lower the knees down keeping the hips right over the knees with the arms close to the body. Bend the elbows and lower the shoulders to elbow height. If that is too much, bend the elbows just to the place where you can stay for the rest of a long deep exhale, even if you have only lowered an inch. Continue to upward facing dog and then downward facing dog.

Surya Namaskara—Sun Salutations

Surya in Sanskrit means sun—or the source of light—seen as the physical and spiritual essence of the world. *Namaskara*—from *namas*—means to bow or adore.

Though in classic ashtanga yoga, the practice begins with sun salute A and B, I have found that adding an extra warm up before, and a few extra variations to the sun salute B sequence, makes the practice more user friendly for all levels of practitioners.

Most of our practices begin with warm up 1 followed by warm up 2 and then sun salute A, followed by sun salute B, with a few variations. Then we do some standing poses, some floor poses and finish. Let's look at some of the benefits and then define some of the groups of poses we use often.

SOME OF THE BENEFITS OF PRACTICING WARM UPS AND SURYA NAMASKARA

- Warms up the body with both cardio exercise and stretching, and warms up joints and muscles.
- Promotes the flow of energy, lymphatic fluid, and circulation.
- Promotes deepening of the breath and the connection of breath with movements that helps in establishing concentration of mind on the flow of body and breath.
- Warms up and prepares for deeper forward folds and backbends.
- Allows for a sense of connection to the heart as we begin with hands at the heart, and move in a prayer-like sequence. Arms over the head, then bowing down. Try to make this a practice of gratitude and heart opening.

Warm Ups and Sun Salute Sequences

All of the sequences which follow, including the warm ups and the surya namaskara (sun salutes) with their variations, have an image sequence in the yoga practices section below. If you do practice your own sequence, start with warm up 1 and 2, surya A, B1, B3, B4, or B5. This is a pretty solid warm up, and even a full practice on days with very little time. Later we will look at options you can add to this, but this is pretty much my standard beginning.

*WARM UP 1 SEQUENCE

This is the Doron Yoga classic warm up 1 sequence. However, you can modify it some according to how you feel. Maybe you do the knee to nose with the back knee on the ground, or maybe you do this with no vinyasa in between. The important part is that you move slowly and allow the body to wake up in a fluid way. (**fig. 145, opposite page**)

- Cat/cow for five deep breaths (bidalasana—bitilasana)

- Hip rotations on all fours, a few to each side (delicious pose)

- Downward facing puppy (uttana shishosana)

- Downward facing dog (adho mukha svanasana)

- Take your right leg up to the sky. Bend the right knee and take it up towards the sky, bringing your right heel to the left side. Stack your hips over each other and thus open the hips. Stay for three deep breaths.

- Inhale, straighten the right leg behind you, and exhale, shift forward, bringing the shoulders over the wrists and the knee to the nose, curling in the belly. Repeat two more times or bring the right knee to the left elbow and back to the sky, then the right knee to the outside of the right elbow and back to the sky.

- Exhale and bring your right foot forward between the hands. If it doesn't reach there, help yourself by using the right hand to bring the foot forward. Come into low lunge (anjaneyasana) for five breaths.

- Step back to plank and take a vinyasa.

- Inhale and take your left leg up to the sky. Bend the left knee and take it up towards the sky and your left heel to the right side. Stack your hips over each other, thus opening the hips. Stay for three deep breaths.

- Inhale and straighten the leg behind you. Exhale and shift forward, bringing the shoulders over the wrists and bringing the knee to the nose, curling in the belly. Repeat two more times or bring the left kneeto the right elbow and back to the sky, and then bring the left knee to the outside of the left elbow and back to the sky.

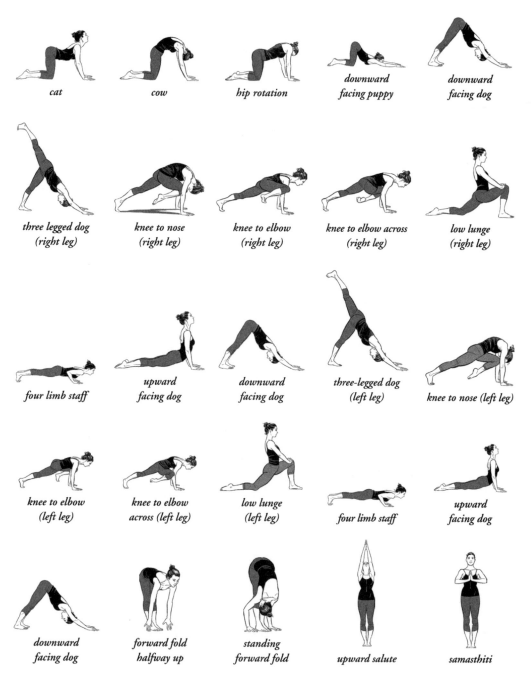

Figure 145, Warm Up Sequence 1 (left to right, top to bottom)

cat   *cow*   *hip rotation*   *downward facing puppy*   *downward facing dog*

three legged dog (right leg)   *knee to nose (right leg)*   *knee to elbow (right leg)*   *knee to elbow across (right leg)*   *low lunge (right leg)*

four limb staff   *upward facing dog*   *downward facing dog*   *three-legged dog (left leg)*   *knee to nose (left leg)*

knee to elbow (left leg)   *knee to elbow across (left leg)*   *low lunge (left leg)*   *four limb staff*   *upward facing dog*

downward facing dog   *forward fold halfway up*   *standing forward fold*   *upward salute*   *samasthiti*

- Exhale and bring the left foot forward between the hands. If it doesn't reach there, help yourself by using the left hand to bring the foot forward. Come into low lunge (anjaneyasana) for five breaths.

- Step back and take a vinyasa.

- Walk the feet to the front of the mat and fold forward (uttanasana).

- Slowly bend the knees and inhale; come all the way up to standing with the arms over the head (urdhva hastasana).

- Exhale and close the hands back to the heart (tadasana or samasthiti).

*Warm-Up 2 Sequence

The main addition here is the high lunge pose—an important preparation for the warrior 1 that follows in most sequences. You can do the entire warm up 2 sequence, or you can simply go to the high lunge after the last downward dog of the warm up 1, and do it on both sides before coming up to mountain pose. (**fig. 146, opposite page**)

- Come to mountain pose (tadasana or samasthiti).

- Inhale; take the hands up over the head (urdhva hastasana).

- Exhale; fold forward (uttanasana).

- Inhale; lengthen halfway up (ardha uttanasana).

- Exhale; take the right foot back. Step the left foot back and go through your vinyasa.

- Inhale; bring the right foot forward between the hands, slowly coming up to crescent high lunge. Hold for five breaths (anjaneyasana). Exhale; bring the hands to the heart (tadasana or samasthiti). Inhale; take the hands up over the head (urdhva hastasana).

- Take your hands to the earth. Step the left foot forward and lengthen the spine halfway up (ardha uttanasana).

- Exhale; fold forward (uttanasana).

- Inhale; come all the way up with hands over the head (urdhva hastasana).

- Exhale; bring the hands to the heart (tadasana or samasthiti).

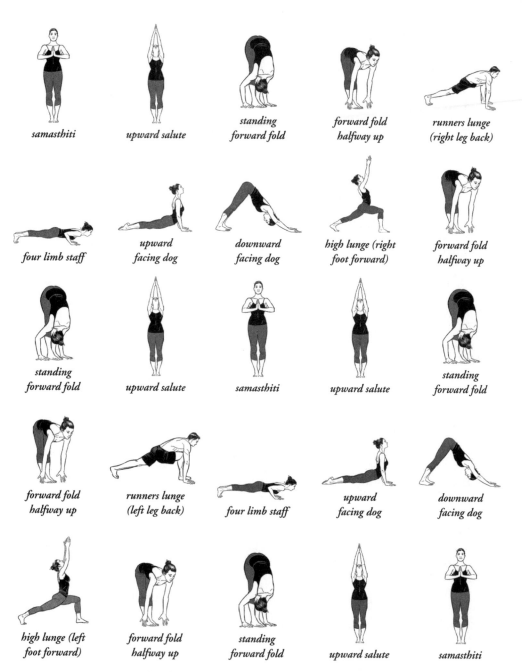

samasthiti

upward salute

standing forward fold

forward fold halfway up

runners lunge (right leg back)

four limb staff

upward facing dog

downward facing dog

high lunge (right foot forward)

forward fold halfway up

standing forward fold

upward salute

samasthiti

upward salute

standing forward fold

forward fold halfway up

runners lunge (left leg back)

four limb staff

upward facing dog

downward facing dog

high lunge (left foot forward)

forward fold halfway up

standing forward fold

upward salute

samasthiti

Figure 146, Warm Up Sequence 2 (left to right, top to bottom)

- Inhale; take the hands up over the head (urdhva hastasana).
- Exhale; fold forward (uttanasana).
- Inhale; lengthen halfway up (ardha uttanasana).
- Exhale; take the left foot back. Step the right foot back and go through your vinyasa.
- Exhale; bring the left foot forward between the hands, slowly coming up to crescent high lunge. Hold for five breaths (anjaneyasana).
- Take your hands to the earth. Step the right foot forward and lengthen the spine halfway up (ardha uttanasana).
- Exhale; fold forward (uttanasana).
- Inhale; come all the way up with hands over the head (urdhva hastasana).
- Exhale; bring the hands to the heart (tadasana or samasthiti).

*Surya Namaskara A (Sun Salute A) Sequence

This is the classic surya A sequence of the ashtanga vinyasa system. (**fig. 147, opposite page)**

- Come to mountain pose (tadasana or samasthiti).
- Inhale; take the arms up over the head (urdhva hastasana).
- Exhale; fold forward (uttanasana).
- Inhale; lengthen halfway up (ardha uttanasana).
- Exhale; step or jump back into low plank and take your vinyasa. Breathe for five deep breaths in downward facing dog (adho mukha svanasana).
- Look between your hands; inhale and step or jump forward, lengthening halfway up as you land (ardha uttanasana).
- Exhale; fold forward over the legs (uttanasana).
- Inhale; come all the way up with the hands over head (urdhva hastasana).
- Exhale and bring the hands to the heart (tadasana or samasthiti).

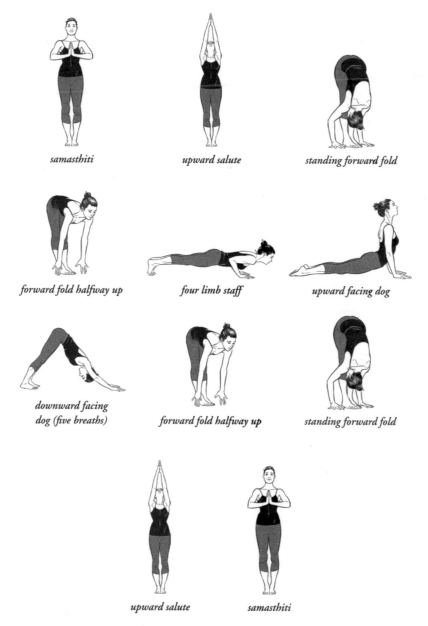

samasthiti *upward salute* *standing forward fold*

forward fold halfway up *four limb staff* *upward facing dog*

*downward facing
dog (five breaths)* *forward fold halfway up* *standing forward fold*

upward salute *samasthiti*

Figure 147, Surya Namaskara A (Sun Salute A)
Sequence (left to right, top to bottom)

*Surya Namaskara B (Sun Salute B) Sequence

This is the classic surya B sequence of the ashtanga vinyasa system. (**fig. 148, opposite page**)

- Bend the knees deeply, lower your hips, and inhale; open your heart and raise your arms up to fierce pose (utkatasana).

- Exhale; fold forward (uttanasana).

- Inhale; lengthen halfway up (ardha uttanasana).

- Exhale; step or jump back, and take your vinyasa.

- From downward dog, bring your right foot forward and rotate the left heel down. Come up into warrior 1 (virabhadrasana I).

- Exhale; lower the hands to the earth. Step the right foot back and go through your vinyasa.

- Bring your left foot forward and rotate the right heel down. Come up into warrior 1 (virabhadrasana I).

- Exhale; lower the hands to the earth. Step the left foot back and go through your vinyasa.

- Take five deep breaths in downward facing dog (adho mukha svanasana).

- Look between your hands, inhale, step or jump forward, and lengthen halfway up (ardha uttanasana).

- Exhale; fold forward (uttanasana).

- Bend the knees deeply, lower your hips, and inhale; open your heart and raise your arms up (utkatasana).

- Exhale; return to mountain pose (tadasana or samasthiti).

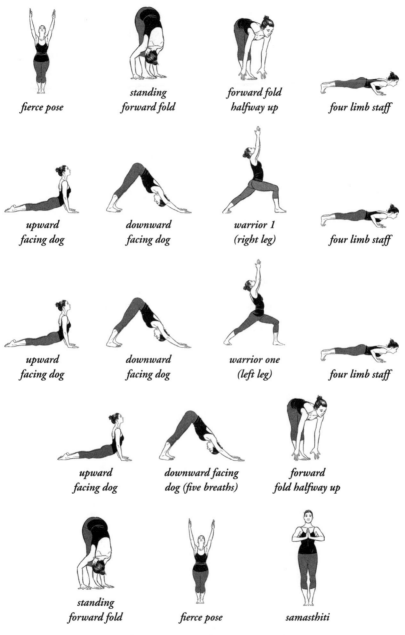

**Figure 148, Surya Namaskara B (Sun Salute B)
Sequence (left to right, top to bottom)**

Surya Nasmaskara Variations

All the variations that follow begin with coming into warrior 1 on the right side, then taking the variation. After taking the variation, lower down to take a vinyasa and repeat on the left side.

You can take five breaths in downward dog once you finish the second side, and either continue to another variation, or make your way back to standing. When I have time and feel strong, I return to standing between the variations, but many times, I just go from one variation to the next with a few breaths in downward dog between them.

The flexitarian method would be to return to standing after surya B1 for example, but skip coming back to standing on the next variation. Always finding the middle way.

*Surya Namaskara B, Variation 1, Twisted Warrior 1 (Surya B1)

This sequence is almost the same as the classical surya B, but with an added twist—great for releasing the spine and moving energy. There are no twists in the ashtanga sun salutes, and since my body was craving one to wake up the spine early on, this has now become a new classic. **(fig. 149, opposite page)**

- From warrior 1, take the twisted warrior variation. Take your left hand forward to the right thigh and your right arm down to the right side on the back leg.

- Twist to the right side, keeping the torso tall and perpendicular to the floor and the right knee bending deeply. Keep rotating your right shoulder to the right, and let your head follow. Hold for five deep breaths.

- Return to warrior 1.

- Lower the arms down to the mat and take your vinyasa.

- Repeat on the left side.

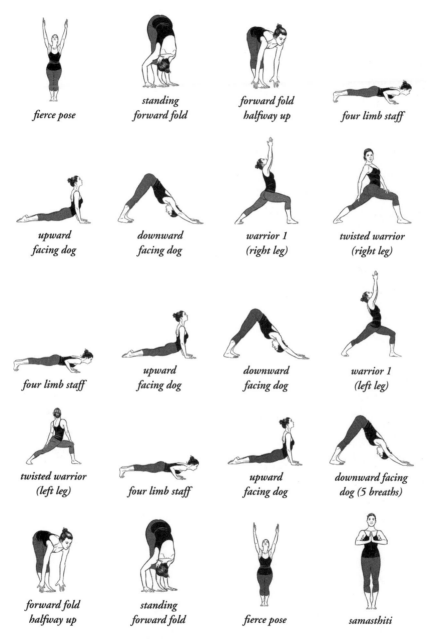

Figure 149, Surya Namaskara B, Variation 1,
Twisted Warrior 1 (Surya B1) (left to right, top to bottom)

*Surya Namaskara B, Variation 2, Shoulder and Hip Opener (Surya B2)

A sequence that opens the shoulders and hips—a great way to warm up quickly and prepare for what is next. On days with less time, I do this on the same round of warriors as surya B1. So it is a B1—B2 combo. (**fig. 150, opposite page**)

- From warrior 1, release your hands down and clasp your fingers behind your back. Lengthen in the spine and move your torso up and back while you take your arms away from the body so that you are creating a gentle backbend.

- Exhale, take your head to the inside of the right knee towards the floor with the arms following, reaching overhead. You are now in humble warrior pose. Hold for five deep breaths.

- With super strong legs and your core engaged, lift all the way back up into warrior 1.

- Exhale and take the hands back down to the floor. Go through a vinyasa.

- Repeat on the left side.

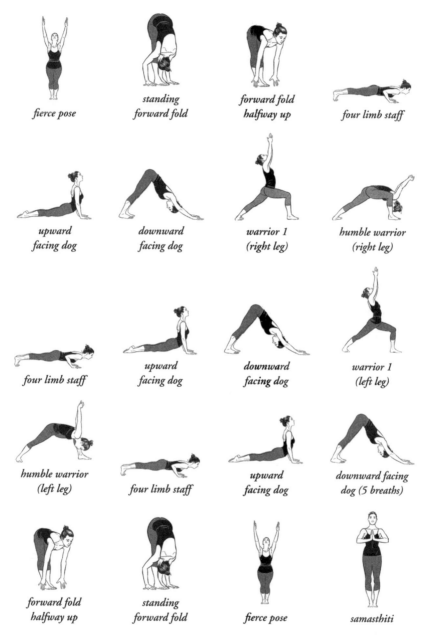

fierce pose

standing
forward fold

forward fold
halfway up

four limb staff

upward
facing dog

downward
facing dog

warrior 1
(right leg)

humble warrior
(right leg)

four limb staff

upward
facing dog

downward
facing dog

warrior 1
(left leg)

humble warrior
(left leg)

four limb staff

upward
facing dog

downward facing
dog (5 breaths)

forward fold
halfway up

standing
forward fold

fierce pose

samasthiti

Figure 150, Surya Namaskara B, Variation 2,
Shoulder and Hip Opener (Surya B2) (left to right, top to bottom)

*Surya Namaskara B, Variation 3, Eagle Arms and Hips (Surya B3)

I know I'm not supposed to have favorites, but if I did, this would be one of them. Opening the shoulders, a bit of backbending, and then a very delicious hip opener—a fantastic way to prepare for the challenging poses that will come ahead. (**fig. 151, opposite page**)

- From warrior 1, take your right arm underneath the left and wrap it around so that the right palm faces the left palm. If it does not quite happen, you might be able to hook your thumbs, and that is fine.

- Lift in the belly, lengthen the spine, and begin going into a backbend while lifting the elbows. Let your gaze go up towards the hands. Keep the right knee bent and hold for five breaths. Inhale and come back up into warrior 1.

- Exhale and bring the hands to the inside of the right foot. Lower the back knee to the ground, untuck the back toes, and either stay here or lower the forearms to a block or to the floor. This is utthana pristhasana (lizard pose).

- Stay and breathe for eight deep breaths.

- Come back to your hands, step the right foot back and take your vinyasa.

- Repeat on the left side.

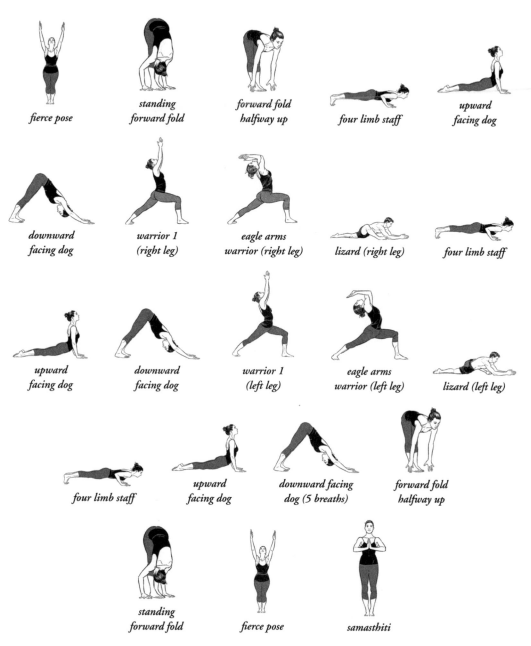

fierce pose

standing
forward fold

forward fold
halfway up

four limb staff

upward
facing dog

downward
facing dog

warrior 1
(right leg)

eagle arms
warrior (right leg)

lizard (right leg)

four limb staff

upward
facing dog

downward
facing dog

warrior 1
(left leg)

eagle arms
warrior (left leg)

lizard (left leg)

four limb staff

upward
facing dog

downward facing
dog (5 breaths)

forward fold
halfway up

standing
forward fold

fierce pose

samasthiti

Figure 151, Surya Namaskara B, Variation 3,
Eagle Arms and Hips (Surya B3) (left to right, top to bottom)

*Surya Namaskara B, Variation 4, Triangle (Surya B4)

This sequence incorporates some classics into one flow. From warrior 1 we move slowly as in meditation with great focus to warrior 2, opening our hips, and continuing with external rotation hip poses to the reverse warrior and triangle. A foundation for most vinyasa classes. (fig. 152, opposite page)

- From warrior 1, open slowly into warrior 2 and hold for two to five deep breaths.

- Turn the right palm up and reverse the warrior. Hold for three deep breaths.

- Come back up through warrior 2, straighten the front leg and come into triangle pose. (You can do extended side angle instead.) Hold for five deep breaths.

- With super strong legs and a lift in the belly, inhale back up to warrior 2.

- Exhale, cartwheel the hands down and take your vinyasa.

- Repeat on the left side.

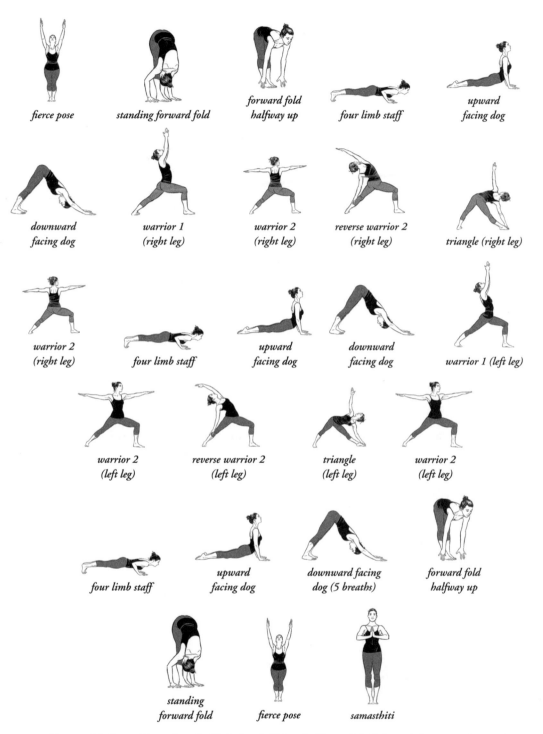

Figure 152, Surya Namaskara B, Variation 4, Triangle (Surya B4) (left to right, top to bottom)

*Surya Namaskara B, Variation 5, Extended Side Angle, Triangle, and Half-Moon (Surya B5)

This is a sequence similar to surya B4 with a few extra poses. You can always do the surya B4 on days with less time or energy. **(fig. 153, pages 225–226)**

- From warrior 1, open slowly into warrior 2 and hold for two to five deep breaths.
- Turn the right palm up and reverse the warrior. Hold for three deep breaths.
- Come back up through warrior 2 and into extended side angle. Hold for five deep breaths.
- With super strong legs and a lift in the belly, inhale back up to warrior 2.
- Straighten your front leg and reach forward for triangle. Hold triangle for three to five breaths.
- Shift the weight forward onto the front leg, keeping the heart open. Raise your back leg into half-moon and hold for five breaths. The bottom hand can be at the floor, on a block or even at your heart.
- Return to warrior 2.
- Exhale, cartwheel the hands down to the floor, and take your vinyasa.
- Repeat on left side.

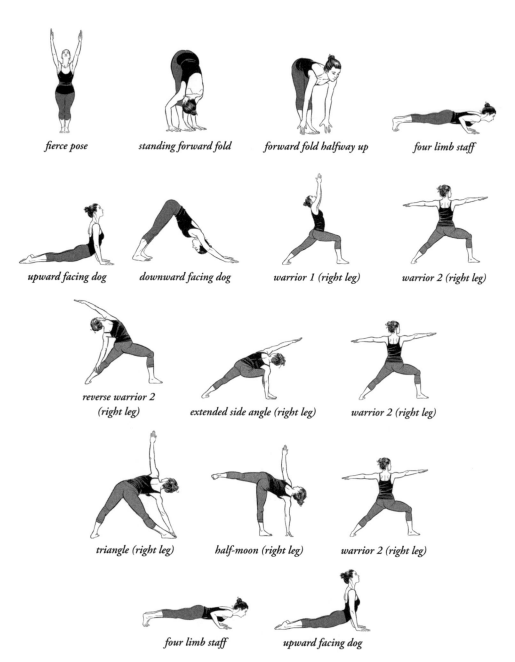

fierce pose standing forward fold forward fold halfway up four limb staff

upward facing dog downward facing dog warrior 1 (right leg) warrior 2 (right leg)

reverse warrior 2
(right leg) extended side angle (right leg) warrior 2 (right leg)

triangle (right leg) half-moon (right leg) warrior 2 (right leg)

four limb staff upward facing dog

Figure 153, Surya Namaskara B, Variation 5, Extended Side Angle, Triangle, and Half-Moon
(Surya B5) (left to right, top to bottom) (cont. next page)

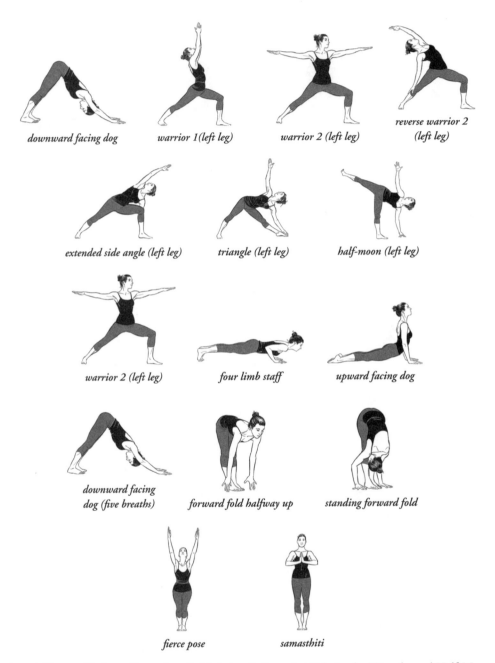

downward facing dog *warrior 1(left leg)* *warrior 2 (left leg)* *reverse warrior 2 (left leg)*

extended side angle (left leg) *triangle (left leg)* *half-moon (left leg)*

warrior 2 (left leg) *four limb staff* *upward facing dog*

downward facing dog (five breaths) *forward fold halfway up* *standing forward fold*

fierce pose *samasthiti*

(cont.) Figure 153, Surya Namaskara B, Variation 5, Extended Side Angle, Triangle, and Half-Moon (Surya B5) (left to right, top to bottom)

Yoga Practices

Time to get to work! There are a variety of sequences offered here for different levels and durations. In reality, you can choose any of these sequences and modify them to your level or needs for the specific day and time you are practicing.

For example, you can walk forward and back (instead of jumping) when doing your warm up, and even skip the vinyasas if necessary. You can also add more vinyasas or take a second chaturanga after upward facing dog, if you need more power and aerobic work.

I did not mention all the vinyasa options, but you can take a vinyasa after each pose if you like. Remember that kapha dominant people may be tempted to skip the vinyasa, though they shouldn't, and pitta dominant people may want to do more of them, even when they have actually had enough. Find your balance.

Most poses offered here have modification options in the asana descriptions, so at first learn what is right for you, and when the practice gets easier, begin doing the full poses. For example, I may have a figure of a supine twist with legs crossed. You may need to take the more basic variation of legs uncrossed. The modifications are shown in the pose description section.

All vinyasa flow sequence poses are to be held for five to eight deep breathes unless otherwise noted or when part of the vinyasa or sun salutes, where you move at a pace of one breath per movement.

Begin each practice with a sit for two minutes to breathe and set an intention. Consider chanting Ohm or another chant. Close each practice with legs up the wall or savasana. Enjoy savasana for at least three minutes, and if you have the time, stay for five to ten minutes. Do not skip it!

For your full practice, either follow one of the set sequences offered in the Doron Yoga practice sequences, or build your own practice according to the Doron Yoga building blocks.

The Doron Yoga Building Blocks

There are eighteen building blocks in the Doron Yoga system. Each block may vary in the number of poses it contains and the amount of flexibility to change the poses in it. The warm ups are pretty set, but you can change how you get in and out of them, as well as add warm up poses or eliminate vinyasas.

The surya namaskara B block may have any combination of the variety of surya B options.

Below you will find the main blocks with optional poses and what to choose according to a basic class (level 1–2) or an intermediate class (level 2–3). All level classes are more or less level 1–2 with more options from the level 2–3. You will have to determine according to your body and the specific day of practice; some days you may feel more of a yoga ninja, and others more like a beginner. Respect your body.

DETAILS OF THE DORON YOGA BUILDING BLOCKS

1. *Opening: intention, meditation, chant*

2. *Warm up 1 and 2*

3. *Surya namaskara A*

4. *Surya namaskara B and/or B1*

5. *Surya namaskara B2 or B3*

6. *Surya namaskara B4 or B5*
   - Level 1–2—surya B1, surya B2, surya B4
   - Level 2–3—surya B, surya B1, surya B3, surya B5

7. *Standing forward fold*
   - All levels—uttanasana (standing forward fold), hold elbows or any other arm variation that feels good for you

8. *Prasarita (wide leg forward fold)*
   - Level 1–2—prasarita A or C
   - Level 2–3—prasarita C then A, with optional sirsasana B (tripod headstand)

9. *Parsvottanasana (pyramid)*
   - Level 1–2—parsvottanasana or parivrtta parsvakonasana modified (revolved extended side angle)
   - Level 2–3—parsvottanasana, parivrtta trikonasana (revolved extended side angle), parivrtta parsvakonasana (revolved extended side angle)

10. *Standing balancing poses*
    - All levels—tree pose, galavasana prep, natarajasana (dancer)

11. *Play time (core, arm balances, and inversions)*
    - All levels core—navasana, bicycle yoga, jatharasana (leg lifts), or core leg twists, side plank
    - Playtime—give yourself some time to play, allow for repeated tries—maybe 2–3 times.
    - Level 1–2—bakasana (crow), dolphin, headstand, handstand prep (L shape)
    - Level 2–3—bakasana (crow), handstand, pincha mayurasana (peacock), sirsasana B (tripod headstand)

12. *On the belly*
    - All levels—salabhasana (locust), baby cobra, sphinx, shoulder stretch, ardha bhekasana (half frog), dhanurasana (bow)

13. *Deep stretch*
    - These can go anywhere you need a break.
    - All levels—thread the needle, pigeon, extended leg supine stretch, or splits

14. *Backbends*
    - Level 1–2—bridge with optional urdhva dhanurasana (upward facing bow)
    - Level 2–3—urdhva dhanurasana (upward bow), eka pada raj kapotasana (king pigeon), natarajasana (full dancer)

15. *Twists, hips, and forward folds*
    - All levels—start with any twist to release the back (on the back or seated)
    - Optional happy baby—can feel great too

- All levels—baddha konasana (bound angle), upavishta konasana (seated wide leg stretch), janu sirsasana A (seated forward fold over one leg), marichyasana C (seated twist), trianga mukha eka pada paschimottanasana (three limbs facing one foot), paschimottanasana (seated forward fold over both legs), and any other basic calming seated poses

16. *Inversions*
    - All levels—baddha konasana (bound angle), upavishta konasana (seated wide leg stretch), janu sirsasana A (seated forward fold over one leg), marichyasana C (seated twist), trianga mukha eka pada paschimottanasana (three limbs facing one foot), paschimottanasana (seated forward fold over both legs), and any other basic calming seated poses
    - Optional sirsasana (headstand) with balasana (child's pose) as release
    - For easy days or when on your cycle, practice viparita karani (legs up the wall)

17. *Meditation, savasana, and closing*
    - All levels—optional supine (on the back) twists, savasana (final relaxation), optional pranayama (breath work)
    - Meditation, set intention, chant, feel gratitude

More practices and pose descriptions in text and video formats can be found on my website: www.doronyoga.com.

Doron Yoga Practice Sequences

The sequences offered here are sample practices of different lengths and different levels of difficulty. You can add and change these sequences as needed. For example, you can use the forty-five minutes, all-levels practice as a base, and then add to it extra hip openers, forward folds, or standing balancing poses. You can also modify levels. If there is an advanced practice you like, such as the seventy-five minutes advanced, you can skip some of the challenging poses, or practice the preparation for them.

These sequences can be practiced over and over, as they are balanced practices. Try to work on doing some of the longer ones as well. After you get comfortable with them, use the guidelines in the Doron Yoga building blocks to create your own variations. Most importantly—breathe and enjoy!

30 Minutes Doron Yoga Vinyasa—Beginners

This is a great quick practice for beginners or those that want a short practice with extra stretching and less movement. This is also a great supplement if you already did other cardio or as an afternoon second practice. (**fig. 154, next page**)

30 Minutes Doron Yoga Vinyasa—All Levels

A quick practice that is good for all. Great for days with less time, but do try and also practice the longer versions of 75 and 90 minutes. (**fig. 155, page 233**)

45 Minutes Doron Yoga Vinyasa—All Levels

Here is another great short/medium practice. It is great for all, as well as for days with less time, or as supplement for cardio. (**fig. 156, page 234**)

45 Minutes Doron Yoga Vinyasa—Advanced

Get to work! This is a no-nonsense, intense 45–minutes practice. If you know your poses, and are ready to dive in, this is for you. Of course you can modify and do the preparation for many of these poses, but if you are new, this may be too much for now. (**fig. 157, page 235**)

60 Minutes Doron Yoga Vinyasa—Beginners

An hour-long yoga practice that is great not only for beginners, but for days when you would rather stretch more and take it easy. If you feel stressed or out of balance with your pitta (fire body type), consider this as a good choice. (**fig. 158, page 236**)

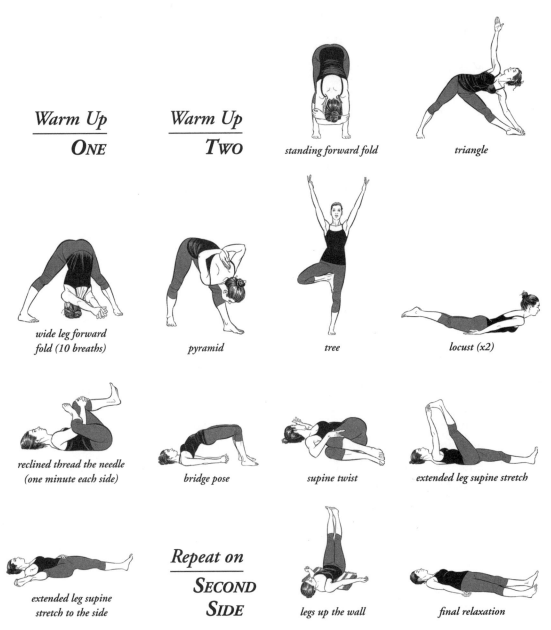

Warm Up
ONE

Warm Up
TWO

standing forward fold

triangle

wide leg forward
fold (10 breaths)

pyramid

tree

locust (x2)

reclined thread the needle
(one minute each side)

bridge pose

supine twist

extended leg supine stretch

extended leg supine
stretch to the side

Repeat on
SECOND
SIDE

legs up the wall

final relaxation

Figure 154, 30 Minutes Doron Yoga Vinyasa—Beginners (left to right, top to bottom)

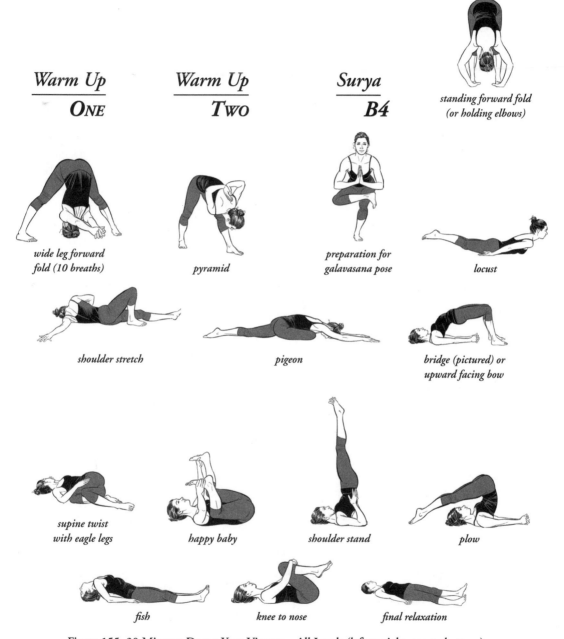

Warm Up
___
ONE

Warm Up
___
TWO

Surya
___
B4

standing forward fold
(or holding elbows)

wide leg forward
fold (10 breaths)

pyramid

preparation for
galavasana pose

locust

shoulder stretch

pigeon

bridge (pictured) or
upward facing bow

supine twist
with eagle legs

happy baby

shoulder stand

plow

fish

knee to nose

final relaxation

Figure 155, 30 Minutes Doron Yoga Vinyasa—All Levels (left to right, top to bottom)

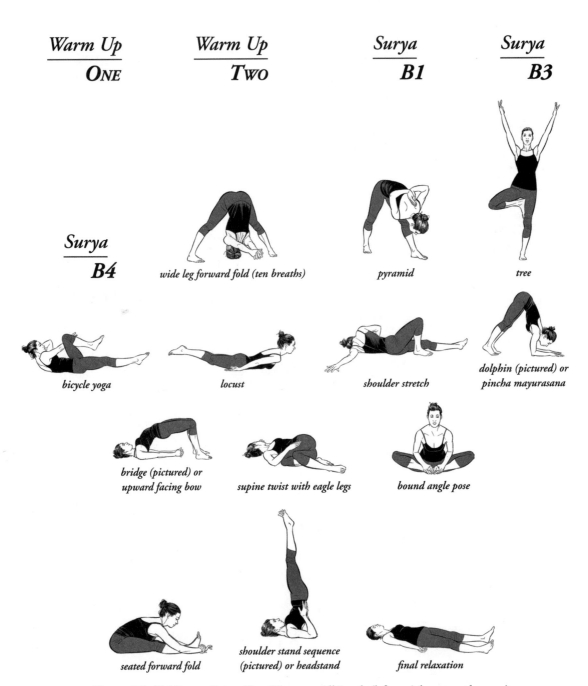

Warm Up ONE

Warm Up TWO

Surya B1

Surya B3

Surya B4

wide leg forward fold (ten breaths)

pyramid

tree

bicycle yoga

locust

shoulder stretch

dolphin (pictured) or pincha mayurasana

bridge (pictured) or upward facing bow

supine twist with eagle legs

bound angle pose

seated forward fold

shoulder stand sequence (pictured) or headstand

final relaxation

Figure 156, 45 Minutes Doron Yoga Vinyasa—All Levels (left to right, top to bottom)

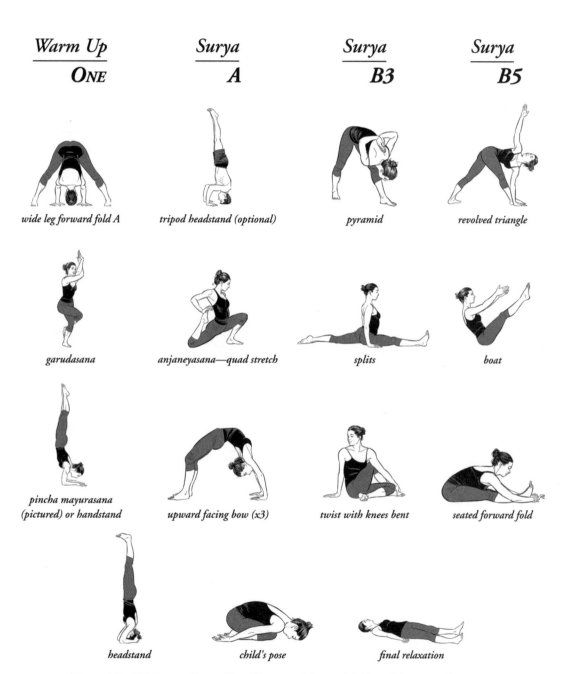

Warm Up	Surya	Surya	Surya
ONE	**A**	**B3**	**B5**

wide leg forward fold A   tripod headstand (optional)   pyramid   revolved triangle

garudasana   anjaneyasana—quad stretch   splits   boat

pincha mayurasana (pictured) or handstand   upward facing bow (x3)   twist with knees bent   seated forward fold

headstand   child's pose   final relaxation

Figure 157, 45 Minutes Doron Yoga Vinyasa—Advanced (left to right, top to bottom)

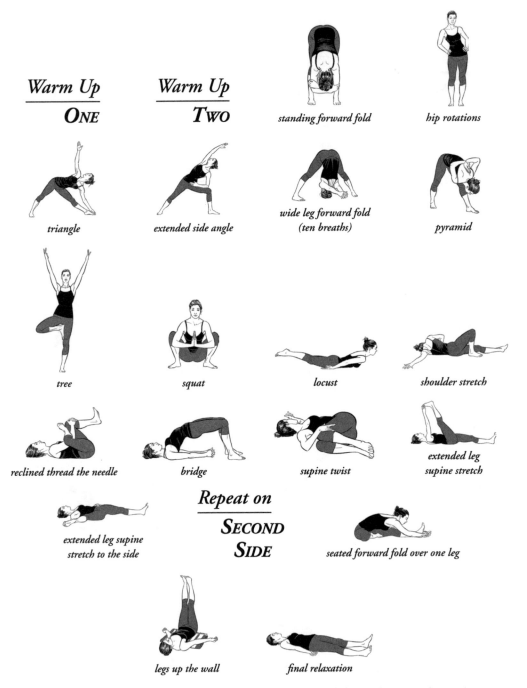

standing forward fold

hip rotations

triangle

extended side angle

wide leg forward fold
(ten breaths)

pyramid

tree

squat

locust

shoulder stretch

reclined thread the needle

bridge

supine twist

extended leg
supine stretch

extended leg supine
stretch to the side

Repeat on
SECOND
SIDE

seated forward fold over one leg

legs up the wall

final relaxation

Figure 158, 60 Minutes Doron Yoga Vinyasa—Beginners (left to right, top to bottom)

60 Minutes Doron Yoga Vinyasa—All Levels

One hour of all the important poses. Though this is a complete practice, try to also do the 75– and 90–minutes all levels sometimes. They offer more depth and additional poses such as core work. (**fig. 159, next page**)

75 Minutes Doron Yoga Vinyasa—All Levels

This practice may be the most useful. You can switch the camel with upward facing bow for variety, and switch the boat pose with bicycle yoga. Or simply alternate this practice with the 90–minutes all levels. (**fig. 160, page 239**)

75 Minutes Doron Yoga Vinyasa—Advanced

A fun flowing practice, with changing poses such as handstands and standing splits. Not for beginners. A great practice for days when you have energy and ready to play. (**fig. 161, pages 240–241**)

90 Minutes Vinyasa Yoga—All Levels

This may be one of the most useful practices. It is complete, long, and offers a great variety of poses. You can substitute the bridge/upward facing bow with camel pose some days. Or alternate this practice with the 75–minutes all levels. (**fig. 162, pages 242–243**)

90 Minutes Doron Yoga Vinyasa—Advanced

This is a master class—challenging and long—that works the entire body with some advanced poses. You can modify these to work with intermediate students as well. Skip some advanced poses, or modify them to work with your level. (**fig. 163, pages 244–245**)

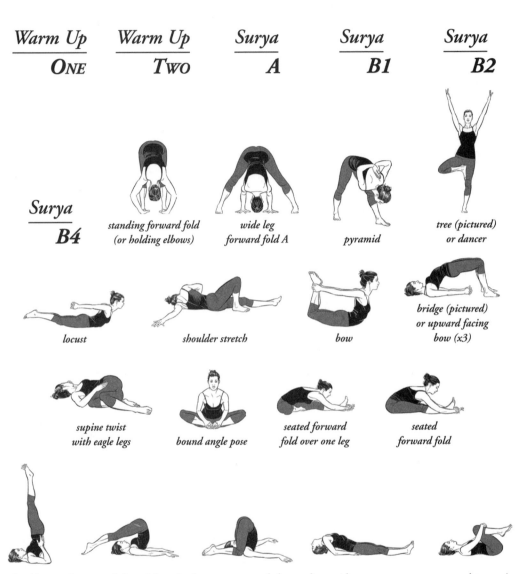

| Warm Up ONE | Warm Up TWO | Surya A | Surya B1 | Surya B2 |

Surya B4

standing forward fold (or holding elbows) · wide leg forward fold A · pyramid · tree (pictured) or dancer

locust · shoulder stretch · bow · bridge (pictured) or upward facing bow (x3)

supine twist with eagle legs · bound angle pose · seated forward fold over one leg · seated forward fold

shoulder stand sequence (left to right: salamba sarvangasana, halasana, karnapidasana, matsyasana, vayu muktyasana)

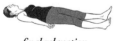

final relaxation

Figure 159, 60 Minutes Doron Yoga Vinyasa—All Levels (left to right, top to bottom)

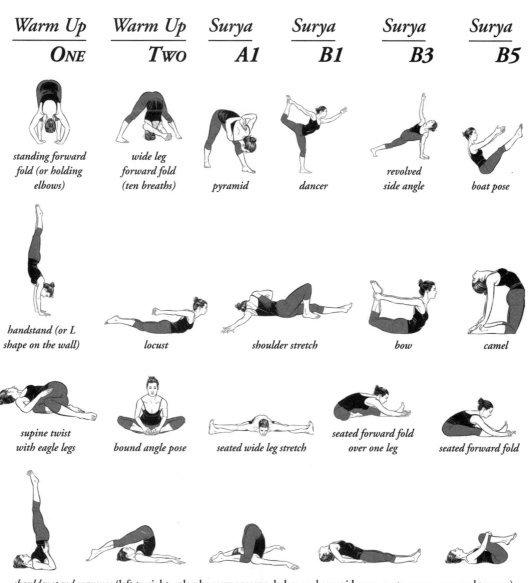

Warm Up ONE	Warm Up TWO	Surya A1	Surya B1	Surya B3	Surya B5

standing forward fold (or holding elbows)

wide leg forward fold (ten breaths)

pyramid

dancer

revolved side angle

boat pose

handstand (or L shape on the wall)

locust

shoulder stretch

bow

camel

supine twist with eagle legs

bound angle pose

seated wide leg stretch

seated forward fold over one leg

seated forward fold

shoulder stand sequence (left to right: salamba sarvangasana, halasana, karnapidasana, matsyasana, vayu muktyasana)

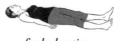

final relaxation

Figure 160, 75 Minutes Doron Yoga Vinyasa—All Levels (left to right, top to bottom)

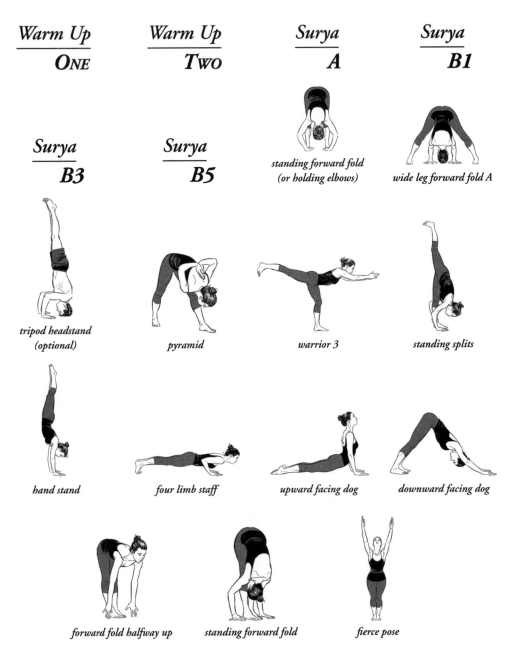

Warm Up
ONE

Warm Up
TWO

Surya
A

standing forward fold
(or holding elbows)

Surya
B1

wide leg forward fold A

Surya
B3

Surya
B5

tripod headstand
(optional)

pyramid

warrior 3

standing splits

hand stand

four limb staff

upward facing dog

downward facing dog

forward fold halfway up

standing forward fold

fierce pose

Figure 161, 75 Minutes Doron Yoga Vinyasa—Advanced (left to right, top to bottom) (cont. next page)

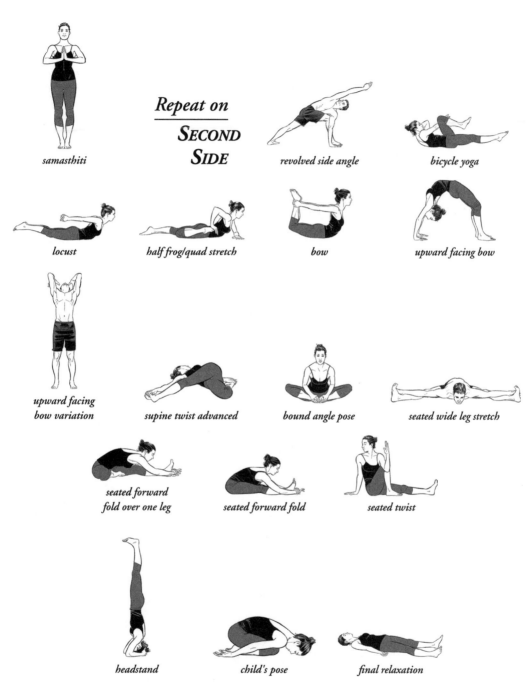

samasthiti

Repeat on
**SECOND
SIDE**

revolved side angle

bicycle yoga

locust

half frog/quad stretch

bow

upward facing bow

*upward facing
bow variation*

supine twist advanced

bound angle pose

seated wide leg stretch

*seated forward
fold over one leg*

seated forward fold

seated twist

headstand

child's pose

final relaxation

(cont.) Figure 161, 75 Minutes Doron Yoga Vinyasa—Advanced (left to right, top to bottom)

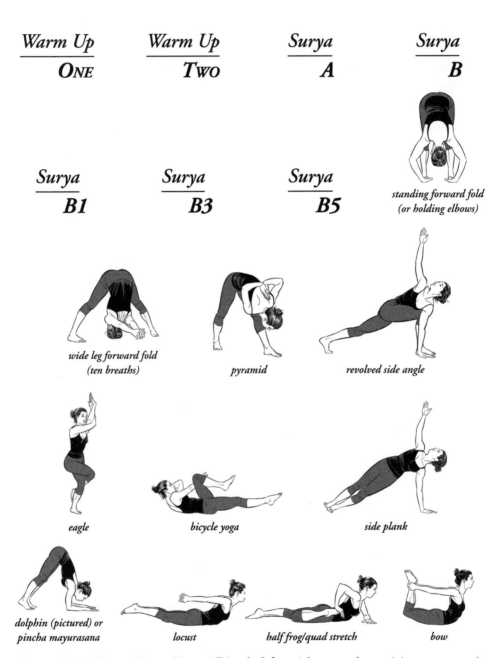

Warm Up ONE	Warm Up TWO	Surya A	Surya B

standing forward fold (or holding elbows)

Surya B1	Surya B3	Surya B5

wide leg forward fold (ten breaths)

pyramid

revolved side angle

eagle

bicycle yoga

side plank

dolphin (pictured) or pincha mayurasana

locust

half frog/quad stretch

bow

Figure 162, 90 Minutes Vinyasa Yoga—All Levels (left to right, top to bottom) (cont. next page)

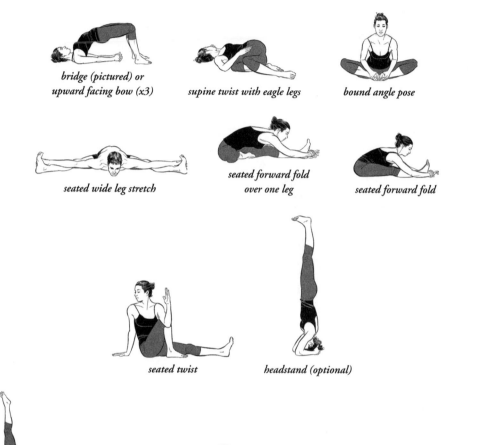

bridge (pictured) or
upward facing bow (x3)

supine twist with eagle legs

bound angle pose

seated wide leg stretch

seated forward fold
over one leg

seated forward fold

seated twist

headstand (optional)

shoulder stand sequence (left to right: salamba sarvangasana, halasana, karnapidasana, matsyasana, vayu muktyasana)

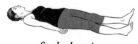

final relaxation

(cont.) Figure 162, 90 Minutes Vinyasa Yoga—All Levels (left to right, top to bottom)

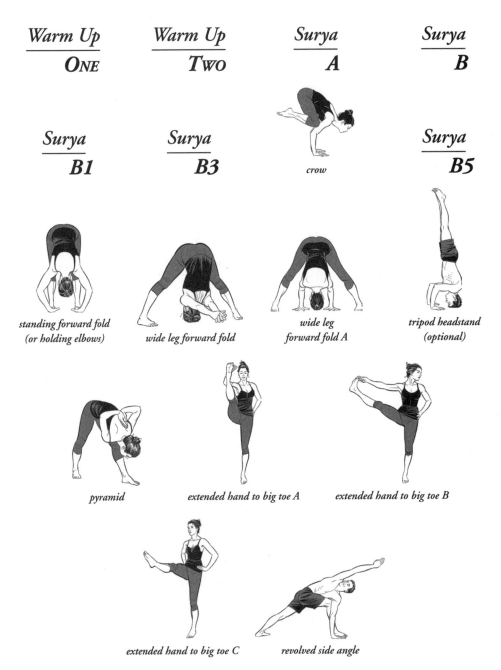

Figure 163, 90 Minutes Doron Yoga Vinyasa—Advanced (left to right, top to bottom) (cont. next page)

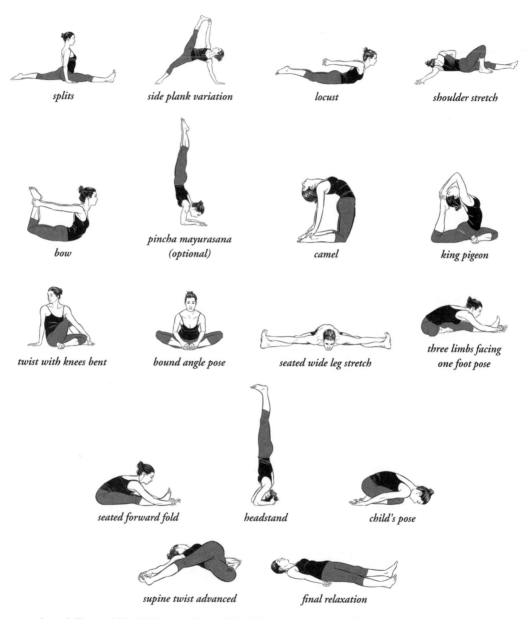

splits

side plank variation

locust

shoulder stretch

bow

pincha mayurasana
(optional)

camel

king pigeon

twist with knees bent

bound angle pose

seated wide leg stretch

three limbs facing
one foot pose

seated forward fold

headstand

child's pose

supine twist advanced

final relaxation

(cont.) Figure 163, 90 Minutes Doron Yoga Vinyasa—Advanced (left to right, top to bottom)

Balancing Your Doshas with Asana

All sequences offered here can be used to balance your doshas. To balance vata, practice much more slowly, hold poses longer, and keep the gaze very steady; most deep stretch practices are suitable for this. To balance kapha, take extra sun salutes and vinyasas, practice what is challenging for you, and don't hold poses very long. To balance pitta, soften your practice, breath, and attitude. See the Ayurveda section for further details.

Complementing Yoga

The asana practice of yoga as outlined in this book will give you most of what you need, as far as physical practices. The poses will stretch your body in every direction, and work most of your muscles. You are bearing you own weight over and over in yoga, as well as often having to work against gravity, which helps to maintain healthy bones and tone the muscles.

Most gym machines isolate your muscles and get you strong in very specific areas. Our bodies work in synergy; we use whole groups of muscles together. Yoga poses use many muscles all at once so you may not feel it the way you would when doing squat reps or some other gym training that is more focused on one area, but you will see your body getting toned all around.

If you would like to, you can mix in additional body weight exercise such as pushups, pull-ups, side planks, and other exercises that use your own body and gravity for work. You can do this with your yoga practice or at another time.

As for cardio, the sun salute will give your heart a bit of a workout, and most other challenging poses, such as deep backbends and some inversions, will get your heart rate moving up as well.

With this being said, I would advise you to do some extra cardio and other movement beyond your yoga practice. You do not need to train for a marathon or be a serious bike rider, but you want to be moving often, either as an additional training or through your daily tasks. It will keep you in better shape and have your energy flowing regularly.

There are many ways to get your heart rate up. I'm all about keeping it natural. I love hiking, long walks with short sprints, a bike ride, or a summer swim. Playing Frisbee or volleyball, dancing, and any sport done as a recreational activity are good choices, as well. Whatever you do, make sure you break a sweat. Do something you love, and you will notice you will also be happier.

Another great way to keep moving is simply to do more of life's tasks on your own. Cleaning your home or car, walking to the store instead of driving, carrying your groceries instead of rolling them in a cart, and weeding your garden instead of hiring someone else are all examples. Think of living your life a bit more old school. Be happy when you actually have to do some physical tasks. Think of Karate Kid waxing the cars.

No matter what form of exercise you do, it is important to keep the core slightly in and lifted to support the lower back. Keeping the knees slightly bent is also very important to protect your joints. Practice with delight and to the level where you can still afford a smile.

The Benefits of Exercise

Humans are meant to move. In prehistoric times, and even after, humans were hunters and gatherers who would squat to start a fire, sprint away from danger, or walk long hours as they moved their residences to find a place with more food availability. This movement kept them in shape and supple. Since most of us drive, sit on chairs, and do not need to fetch water from the well, it is good to have some additional exercise practices.

Exercising will make you stronger—muscles will develop to protect your bones and tone your body. Your bones will also get stronger, as they need to resist the pressure put onto them. Moving the joints in a healthy manner helps sustain joint mobility and flexibility. Regular exercise will strengthen your heart and help keep your blood pressure under control, improving your cardio ability. No doubt that the more you use the lungs, and maybe even use them better as you learn pranayama, the better your control of the lungs and respiratory system becomes. This will help keep you young for the long term.

Your digestion will improve as well. Moving helps improve your digestion and your bowel function.

Exercising stimulates the release of endorphins, which improves mood, decreases stress, anxiety, and depression, and gives you an overall good feeling. This may even get addictive, but some "addictions" are good ones. Keep exercising regularly to maintain the natural high it offers. Since exercise increases the feeling of being energetic, light, and powerful, when feeling this high, I do not want to go eat junk food afterward, so it even encourages eating healthier. When you move, your blood flow increases to bring nutrients and oxygen to the entire body, including your brain, so yes, it also helps your mind!

Sleep is also improved, as when you exercise, hormones are released that will later help improve sleep and calmness. Okay, I think we can agree it is good to move!

Some Exercise Options to Complement Yoga

Walking: This is one of my favorites. Walk for a minimum of thirty minutes at a fast pace. Keep your hands moving with your body. Do a two-minute sprint every ten minutes. Try to walk when possible. Do you need to drive? Don't worry about parking far away; the extra walking is good for you.

Swimming: This is fantastic as it both works your heart muscle and tones the whole body. For me it is also a sort of meditation and an opportunity to be absorbed by the water, like being in the womb, but with lots of space to move.

Dancing: I love any form of dancing, especially dances that encourage you to move your whole body in all directions. Some of the greatest dances are done barefoot, have no prescribed form, and allow you to move to your ability. Take a dance class or just go wild in your living room!

Biking: Get your cardio and strengthen your legs. Make sure you keep your spine long and not hunched. If you are going for long rides, try going at your full speed capacity once in a while to exercise your heart and lungs.

Running: A good cardio workout, running also strengthens the legs and glutes. My only hesitation with running is the possible damage to knees and the lower back. If you do decide to make running part of your cardio practice, take the extra time to learn how to do it properly. Keep the knees slightly bent, your body slightly tipping forward, and move each leg forward as if to keep from falling. Keep you lower back long, and try to keep a slight lift in your belly to support your back.

Traditional ways of living: Washing your car, cleaning your home, cleaning your bathtub, and any other work that could be automated or delegated to others can be a source of cardio exercise. You will gain strength, save energy, save money, and enjoy seeing the fruits of your own work.

Women and Yoga

For most of India's history, primarily men practiced yoga. A big shift happened when Indra Devi, an Eastern European woman, asked Krishnamacharya—the grandfather of most yoga practiced today—to teach her yoga. Though he refused at first, her persistence and dedication convinced him to take her under his wing. Indra Devi later took this practice to California, where she taught many celebrities, and eventually to South America, as well.

Now that yoga is at least as popular with women as it is with men (probably even more so), it is important to understand a few specifics related to women practicing yoga.

Yoga and Menstruation

In Mysore, India, at Pattabhi Jois's institute, women are asked to stay home and rest during their menstrual cycle. This is because of the idea that women have less energy during this time of the month and should rest. However, there are many women who actually feel more energized during this time, or at least still have enough energy to practice, either the same way or in a modified, gentler way. Today in the West, most women will still practice during menstruation, though they may stay away from inversions. They may practice poses such as downward facing dog and uttanasana (forward fold), but not poses such as salamba sarvangasana (shoulder stand) or sirsasana (headstand).

There has been much discussion about menstruation and inversion in the yoga world, but there has not been one clear conclusion made. Many teachers caution not to do inversions while menstruating. One fear that has now been disproven was that practicing inversions during menstruation would cause endometriosis. All agree now that inversions are not good for someone that *already* has endometriosis, but inversions do not cause it. If a woman already has endometriosis, then she should avoid inversions while menstruating.

Another problem that may occur if inversions are practiced while a woman is on her cycle is vascular congestion. This is not very common but may happen, especially during the first few days when bleeding is heavier or when inversions are held for more than a minute or two; however, there have not been any studies that confirm this.

In yoga there is an energy called *apana*, which is in charge of elimination and is said to move the energy downward. Some teachers claim that doing inversions during your period interferes with the natural downward flow that is supposed to occur. This interference may cause a temporary stop in the bleeding and heavier bleeding later on.

I have met many women for whom this is not true; they can practice inversions while menstruating and feel fine. If you want to be on the safe side during your heavy bleeding days, either skip full inversions and take legs up the wall, or explore them for a few breaths to see how you feel. Note how you feel a few hours later, as well. In general, it is not such a bad idea to back off sometimes and just take it easy.

PREMENSTRUAL YOGA

Before the menstrual cycle, many women have a variety of PMS symptoms, including irritability, bloating, headaches, and heaviness in the pelvic region. Some get more emotional than usual, and some even experience depression. The body and the mind are connected and affect each other. Yoga can help with these symptoms, but it is important to always listen to the body; you may need to go a bit easier than you normally would.

If you have strong PMS symptoms, instead of a full practice, you may decide to do some reclined poses, such as:

- Supta padangusthasana (reclined hamstring stretch)
- Supta baddha konasana (reclined bound angle pose)
- Gentle reclined twists

Other poses that may feel good are:

- Baddha konasana (bound angle pose)
- Upavishta konasana (seated wide leg stretch)
- Viparita karani (legs up the wall)
- Prasarita padottanasana (wide leg forward fold)
- Adho mukha svanasana (downward dog)
- Bridge pose or supported bridge
- Savasana (corpse pose) reclining on a bolster

Remember that we are all different. An advanced student is someone that knows to listen to his or her body, and feels what is right for them at that specific moment. Practice with awareness, and learn to be sensitive to your body's needs. You are the ultimate judge of what is right for you.

As prehistoric humans, we were moving around, fast and slow, bending, squatting, running, crouching, sprinting, reaching, climbing, and yes, also resting. Today's lifestyle is not natural for our human bodies. Yoga is a great tool to help us move the body in ways that balance out the modern way of living. Yoga and possibly some other physical activities keep you active, stretched, and healthy. This is true for your body, but not less important for your mind, and breath. When we practice yoga, we learn to focus on the breath, deepen it, stretch the lung areas, as well as focus the mind, release tension and stress, and find more peace. The stretching and twisting also helps our digestion, so not only is it important what we eat, but also how we digest. In India there is a folk saying, "You are what you digest"; so yoga and food are good partners.

Being active and practicing yoga is an important part of the flexitarian method, and of course a major part of the yoga lifestyle. Remember to show up. Make it a good habit to show up every day, even if you do just a little bit. Before you know it, you will not be able to live without it.

Next, let us see the sister practice of the yoga poses. Pranayama (breath work) and yoga asana (yoga poses) work synergistically, and support each other in helping you achieve long lasting, sustainable health and joy.

— 5 —

Breath Work—*Pranayama* and Energy Cultivation

N ow that we are moving, stretching, and even breathing deeply with the ujjayi breathing (victorious breath), we can add another layer to our practice to take us deeper. We will add some simple breathing practices (pranayama) that will help us improve our lung capacity, energize and revitalize our life force—our prana, or vital energy—and help us steady the mind and concentration, which is of great help for the meditation practices that will follow.

Pranayama, sometimes called breath control or yogic breathing, offers a variety of practices to help regulate our body and even the mind and our emotions as well as cultivate energy. One of the main books of physical yoga, *The Hatha Yoga Pradipika*, says that when the breath wanders, the mind also is unsteady. But when the breath is calmed, the mind too will be still, and the yogi achieves long life. Therefore, one should learn to control the breath.

Not only will you be healthy now, but practicing pranayama is also one of the best tools for longevity. Most humans start to lose their lung capacity after age thirty, and since we do not breathe fully to begin with (most people only use about 10 percent of their lung capacity), this gets worse with the years. The cells that could be delivering oxygen to vital organs slowly begin to die. With pranayama, we keep our organs alive. Aging also involves losing control of body and mind over the years, which pranayama can help slow down, as pranayama practices help control the body (breathing nutrients into the cells, cultivation of energy) and mind (maintaining focus and alertness).

There are a variety of pranayama practices with different purposes. Some are cooling, some create energy and heat, some may be calming, and others bring about balance and long-term energy. We use the breath to energize the body, cleanse it, relax the mind and become clearer and more focused.

Pranayama can produce very quick results. However, anytime you practice pranayama and feel slightly uncomfortable, please stop immediately. Since these practices also affect our mind, it is important not to push the practice if you feel dizzy, anxious, stressed, or have any other feeling of discomfort. Please consult with your doctor before taking on pranayama practices. This is especially true for pregnant women, people with recent heart conditions, and people who suffer from high blood pressure.

Benefits of *Pranayama*

Physically, pranayama improves the functioning of the digestive system, removes toxins from the body, and improves cardiovascular functioning and circulation, as well as improves functioning of the lungs, which can promote longevity. Pranayama activates the flow of energy in the body, which can help with being more alert and present and may allow you to need less sleep when practiced regularly.

Pranayama complements and improves the physical yoga (asana): kapalabhati helps tone the belly and serves as a nice warm up, while viloma helps expand the lung capacity, deepen the breath, and focus and steady the mind. Sitali can help cool the mind and body if we are overheating, and nadi shodhana can close practice with a balancing and meditative effect.

Many of the pranayama practices soothe the nervous system, release tension and anxiety, calm the body and mind, and help bring emotions into balance. They balance the left and right sides of the brain, helping us further come into a state of balance and harmony, which along with the mind control aspect of pranayama, helps prepare for meditation.

The breath that flows through the nostrils is more than just a physical thing. It is known as the *swara*, breath that contains the life force. Our breath commands the activity of the mind, and when it flows through both nostrils evenly with no distraction, it enables a state of bliss.

Principles of *Pranayama*

Ideally, pranayama *should* be practiced on an empty stomach when we wake up. Some prefer to meditate or do their yoga asana practice first. I find that some pranayama practice before meditation or asana, some after asana, and some before sleep are ideal.

A healthy person should take fifteen breaths per minute, or 21,600 breaths per day. Most people breathe much faster. It is common for people to have shallow breathing and to breathe only from the chest. There is a traditional claim that time is measured by our breath. Thus, if we can slow our breathing, we can slow our aging. Pranayama helps us learn how to control and regulate our breathing. Pranayama (breath work) and physical yoga (asana) both create heat and energy in our body, and support each other in improving our physical and mental health. They are the basics for good mind training and meditation, just like eating well is the foundation for all other practices. Let's see how we can increase the flow of this prana energy.

Preparing for Pranayama

Sit in a comfortable position—cross-legged or on your ankles is normally advised, however any sitting position that allows you to keep your spine tall without too much effort is great. Keep your hips higher than your knees. If this is not possible, or if you have a hard time keeping your spine tall, elevate your seat—a cushion, folded blanket, bolster, or even a chair can work—just make sure to have your spine tall so you have room to breathe!

Practice in a clean room with clean air and no distractions. Take a few ujjayi breaths (victorious breaths) before you begin any other pranayama (breath work) practices.

Pranayama Practices

In the descriptions below I will offer you a variety of techniques and methods of practicing pranayama. Master your ujjayi breathing (victorious breath) first. Learn to use it with your physical yoga practice (asana). Then, learn your deerga swasa (expanding your lungs), which is a great to do at the beginning of your physical yoga practice, as it will expand your breathing capability within your practice.

Later, master nadi shodhana (balancing breath). This can be done anytime, but I love doing it after my physical yoga, as it wraps it all up. Kapalnhati is wonderful to wake up with, or stimulate your physical yoga practice. Anytime you need some more heat or to get started, do a round of kapalbhati (breath of fire). I love doing it at the beginning of my physical yoga practice (asana). From then on you will be able to practice the pranayama of your choice according to your needs.

I offer a progression with different lengths of counting the breath. A count is more or less a second. You may find that at first you count your breath a bit more quickly, but as you get comfortable with the practice—and you will; it is only a matter of time—you will find yourself counting slowly and more calmly.

The more you practice and begin to master some of these practices, the more you will find yourself practicing pranayama. Sometimes you will arrive at a red light and simply observe your ujjayi breath (victorious breath) or do a round of sitali if it is hot outside or kapalabhati if it is cold. You can look forward to having pranayama (breath work) as your best friend.

Ujjayi Breath—Victorious Breath or Throat Breathing

Ujjayi is the basic and most fundamental breath we use in asana practice, but it can be practiced anywhere and anytime. It is nostril breathing that passes through a slightly restricted throat. This creates a soft sound, which helps us stay aware of our breathing and maintain a focused mind. It also allows us to have better control of our breath, as we can breath slower and smoother. Ujjayi (victorious breathing) should flow easily and smoothly without much effort. It should feel like coming home. I practice it every time I get a bit distracted, such as when driving, or as a quick preparation for meditation.

Swasa Breath—Uncontrolled Breath

Swasa breath is a scattered breath or rapid breath, such as you might do when angry. To bring the breath back into balance in this case, practice ujjayi (victorious breath) and hold the exhalation while connecting the mulabandha (root control center) to the ground. This will help ground your energy as well as bring space into the thinking mind, thus creating relief from strong emotions or tension.

Deerga Swasa—Expanding Your Lungs

Deerga swasa is a three-part breathing exercise that helps create space in the lungs so that you can breathe more deeply and smoothly and utilize the maximum lung capacity. It is a great preparation for your physical yoga practice. It is very calming to the mind, creating a sense of control and relaxation. The deep breathing oxygenates and detoxifies the body.

Method of practice: Bring your awareness to the breath, and breathe through the nostrils, keeping the breath soft and deep. Allow a deep exhale to empty the breath from the lungs. Then, as if you were filling a jug where the water begins filling from the bottom, begin your inhale in the belly. This is the first stage. Then bring the breath up into the lower chest and allow your ribcage to expand. This is the second stage. In the third stage, slowly keep breathing up into the upper chest all the way into the collarbones and the back of the body.

Pause briefly with the body full of breath, and then begin exhaling in the reverse order: upper chest, lower chest and lower abdomen. Bring your abdomen in towards the back to complete the exhalation. Keep the spine tall as you exhale and just use the breath to relax the shoulders, jaw, and forehead. Do so without any force or tension. You will find more space as you repeat this. Repeat five times.

- Inhale slowly through the belly, chest, and upper chest
- Exhale slowly and watch the belly, chest, and upper chest; release

Another variation of this is four-part breathing. It is similar to three-part breathing, but we add an emphasis of breathing into the back, which includes the lower back and especially the space between the shoulder blades.

Begin by inhaling into the belly, then up to the lower chest, then to the back, and eventually to the upper chest. This expands the lungs not only all the way from bottom to top, but also front and back. Really focus on bringing the breath into the back of the body. Work on doing this exercise slowly with lots of awareness on every part of the breathing process.

Kumbhaka—Breath Retention

The practice of pranayama involves controlling the way we breathe, the speed of our breath, and which nostril we breathe through, as well as periods of pauses during which we retain (or hold) our breath. BNS Iyengar, one of my Indian teachers, considered the practice of kumbhaka to be the real practice of pranayama, as it is this control of breath—the place where we do not waste our breath—that is the practice of prolonging our life and controlling our mind.

Anytime kumbhaka is offered, make sure you take it only to your comfort level. If you find that you are gasping for air after a round of kumbhaka, please reduce or eliminate it. If you have high blood pressure or are pregnant, avoid the practice of kumbhaka.

Viloma—Three-Part Breathing

Viloma pranayama is deerga swasa with pauses. Make sure you are comfortable with deerga swasa before moving on to viloma. As with deerga swasa, viloma is a great pranayama practice to do before your asana, as it will expand your lungs and help settle the mind.

Method of practice: Exhale completely, and begin your inhale. After you have inhaled a third of the way, pause for two seconds. Inhale another third and pause for two seconds. Inhale all the way, tuck your chin to the throat (jalandhara bandha), and hold for two to five seconds. Release and exhale slowly. Repeat this three times or more. As you practice this pranayama, you will get used to expanding your breath even more. Be sure to practice at a comfortable rate. If after your pause, you find that you are gasping for air, reduce the length of pause time or stay with deerga swasa for now.

The second step is to do the same practice while you exhale. Inhale completely and begin your exhale. After you exhale a third of the way, pause for two seconds. Exhale another third and pause for two seconds. Exhale all the way out, activate mulabandha and uddiyana bandha, and hold for two to five seconds.

The third stage is a combination of the first two stages—taking pauses while inhaling as well as while exhaling. Please, do make sure you are comfortable with each step before progressing onto the next one. This is a fantastic practice that can be done anytime, and it is a great preparation for nadi shodhana as well as yoga asana (physical yoga).

- Inhale a third of the way and pause for two seconds
- Inhale a third more and pause for two seconds
- Inhale all the way and pause for two to five seconds
- Exhale a third of the way and pause for two seconds
- Exhale a third more and pause for two seconds
- Exhale all the way and pause for two to five seconds

Balance Your Brain and Emotions

We have the power to control our brain, mind, emotions, and energies by controlling our breath. Simple practices of breathing through one nostril at a time can help manipulate the energy in our bodies. These are simple practices that can create great change, and help us find balance and reduce stress in a quick way.

Learn about Your Breathing Patterns

Place your fingers underneath both nostrils, and take a few quick sharp exhales. Notice which nostril seems more open, or dominant.

The left nostril represents the moon, the feminine, the abstract, the passive, and the right side of the brain. It is conducive to creating art, meditating, relaxing, and connecting with intuition.

The right nostril represents the sun, the masculine, the analytical, the active and the left side of the brain. It is conducive to active states, such as working, exercising, eating, and making plans.

As you can already imagine, we have the power to control our brain, our mind, and the type of mood we want to be in. Most people breathe through one nostril at a time and switch the nostril only every ninety to one hundred twenty minutes or so.

Our nostril dominance may be influenced by what we do and how we feel. Notice that when you are very hungry, your right nostril is more dominant. When you are sleepy, you may find that your left nostril is dominant. If you like to sleep on your side, notice that when you lie on your right side, you sleep more calmly. Sleeping on the right side allows easier breathing through the left nostril, and thus activates the abstract, spacey right side of the brain, which allows for better sleep.

Learning to read your nostrils will help you be aware of where your head is, and with the control of the breath, you will have the ability to control your mind.

Surya Bedhana—Sun Dominant Breath Control/Right Nostril Breathing

This practice will increase the sun effects—the analytical, masculine, active, thinking mind.

Method of practice: Hand setup—with your right hand open, fold the index and middle fingers in, so you are left with the thumb on one side and the pinky and ring finger on the other. Place your hand on your nose, with the thumb on one side and the pinky and ring finger on the other. The fingers will serve to open and close the nostrils.

Close the left nostril with your right pinky and ring fingers pressing under the bony part of the nose. Breathe slowly and steadily through your right nostril five to twenty-five times. Release, take a few breaths, and repeat as needed.

Breathe through the right nostril only, for five to twenty-five breaths.

Chandra Behdana—Moon Dominant Breath Control/Left Nostril Breathing

This practice will increase the moon effects—the artistic, feminine, passive, abstract mind.

Method of practice: Use the same hand setup as with surya bedhana. Close the right nostril with your right thumb pressing under the bony part of the nose. Breathe slowly and steadily through your left nostril five to twenty-five times. Release, take a few breaths, and repeat as needed.

Breathe through the left nostril only, for five to twenty-five breaths.

Nadi Shodhana—Alternate Nostril Breathing or Balancing Breath

Sometimes known as alternate nostril breathing, *nadi shodhana* is a helpful tool for bringing the body and mind into balance. Classically, it aims at balancing the energies in the body and allowing a powerful flow of energy through the spine to the rest of the body and beyond. On a simple practical level, nadi shodhana is a great tool for balancing our mind and emotions.

There are a variety of teachings that include different ratios or breathing. Some recommend even inhales and exhales, and slowly increasing the length of the kumbhaka (retention). Many aim at reaching the ratio of 1:4:2. This means that the exhalation is twice the length of the inhalation and the kumbhaka is four times the length of the inhalation. For now, all kumbhaka in the nadi shodhana practices will be at the top of the inhalation only. No exhalation kumbhaka for now. Some practice examples are 2:8:4 or 4:16:8.

We will combine the advice of a few teachings (always seeking to maximize the best techniques), and start with no kumbhaka first, and then slowly add it in.

Method of practice: Use the same hand setup as with surya bedhana. Alternate the release of thumb on one side and the pinky and ring finger on the other side to control which nostril is open. We will begin with inhale and twice as long exhales, but with no kumbhaka. Start with 2:4, when easy, move onto 3:6, then to 4:8.

- Inhale through the left for a count of three
- Exhale through the right for a count of six
- Inhale through the right for a count of three
- Exhale through the left for a count of six

This completes one full round. Practice this for six rounds.

Once this is easy move on to practices with kumbhaka.

Since there are a variety of practices with kumbhaka, I recommend starting with 4:4:6. If this is too much lower it to 4:2:6 or even 2:2:4.

Here is an example of progression from easier to harder, but remember to stay with what is good for now even if it is the easiest. No need to rush, and no need to ever achieve the longer practices. You may find that as you meditate more, and practice asana more, your pranayama practices will improve as well.

- Beginners stage: 2:2:4, 4:2:4, 4:2:6, 4:4:6

- Intermediate stage: 4:8:6, 4:8:8, 4:12:8, 4:16:8

- Advanced stage: 6:24:12, 8:32:16

Here is the instruction for practicing 4:4:6. It will be the same for all other options just with different numbers.

- Inhale through the left for a count of four

- Kumbhaka for a count of four

- Exhale through the right for a count of six

- Inhale through the right for a count of four

- Kumbhaka for a count of four

- Exhale through the left for a count of six

Again, only raise the count when it is comfortable, and recognize that not every day will be the same. Some days you will do much better, and others less. That is okay. The important thing is that you show up and practice!

Practice six rounds to begin with, and eventually do twelve rounds each time. You will obviously progress much faster if you do twelve rounds each time you practice. Sure it takes time—so again, it is better to do three rounds than none.

Nadi shodhana is one of the most important practices in this book for your body, mind, and spirit. It is a link between our yoga asana, breath, energy, and mind training. Make sure you practice it at least three times a week for a minimum of three rounds, and ideally four—five times a week for twelve rounds each time.

Kapalabhati—Breath of Fire

Kapalabhati (breath of fire), or the skull-shining breath as it is literally translated, is an invigorating, energizing, heating, and purifying breathing technique. It is a very active, forced exhalation with a passive inhalation.

Do not practice kapalabahti if you are pregnant or menstruating, or if you have high blood pressure or have had recent abdominal surgery, as it is very active in the core area; it creates heat, and can raise the heart rate.

Method of practice: Inhale three-quarters of the way in. Then take sharp exhales through the nose, allowing the inhalation to be passive. The exhalations are done by pressing the lower belly inward, towards the back—or pumping the belly to the back—and thus forcing the air out of the nose. If you are a beginner, please place your hands on your lower belly to help with the pumping motion. It is not easy for everyone to isolate the belly movement at first.

Begin slowly, maybe with one exhalation per second or two. No need to do very quick kapalabhati. It is more important to take a powerful exhale and really move the belly in. You can begin with a round of twenty exhales. Then take a few slow calm breaths and go for another round. Practice two to four rounds.

If this is comfortable enough, consider taking a big inhalation after your last sharp exhale, and do a round of kumbhaka for a count of ten. Then release the breath slowly. Take a restful breath and start again.

Over time, increase the number of exhales in every round. Starting with twenty, then thirty, and maybe fifty. Ultimately, you may increase to one hundred twenty sharp exhales with a kumbhaka of fifteen seconds. Again, this may take years of practice for some, or just a few weeks for others. Some sources recommend not going beyond one hundred twenty exhales per round. The kumbhaka at the end is optional and many schools of yoga do not do it. I find that there is a beautiful feeling of energy running through the body when the kumbhaka is included. Some say they feel "high" while they take the kumbhaka.

- Exhale sharply through the nose
- Inhale passively
- Exhale sharply through the nose and repeat up to one hundred twenty times

- Inhale and take the kumbhaka
- Exhale slowly

This is one practice I do almost daily, either before my asana practice or simply in the morning, as it helps the bodily systems to wake up. Like nadi shodhana (alternate nostril breathing), I recommend practicing this at least three to four times a week, for a minimum of two rounds.

Sitali (Seetali) Pranayama—Cooling Breathing

In the old days, yogis did not cool themselves with external resources; they did not eat ice cream, drink ice water, or turn on the AC. Instead they practiced *sitali pranayama* (cooling breathing) to lower the body temperature. Sitali breathing calms the mind, reduces stress by calming the fight or flight response, and may help to lower blood pressure and calm the nervous system.

Method of practice: Begin by exhaling completely. Curl the tongue between the lips as if you were pretending to be a fish, and then inhale. Allow the air to pass through the curled tongue. Lower the chin and hold the breath (kumbhaka) for a count of ten or however long is comfortable for you. Then exhale slowly and rest for a breath. Repeat six to twelve times.

- Exhale fully
- Inhale through the tongue
- Kumbhaka
- Exhale

Variation: For those who cannot roll the tongue into the curled position, there are two options. The first is to roll the tongue into the mouth, so that it rests on the roof of the mouth. The other option is to practice sitkari (cooling breath 2, below).

Practice sitali especially when hot, or emotionally unbalanced. It is also a great practice for anytime there is inflammation, including asthma, or even to cool down from hot flashes.

Sitkari—Cooling Breath 2

Sitkari is another pranayama that has a cooling effect similar to sitali. When you practice sitkari (cooling breath 2), the air passes through the teeth, rides over the tongue, and cools the body.

Method of practice: Open your lips while keeping your upper and lower teeth touching lightly. Inhale through the mouth with a hissing sound, filling the lungs completely. Then part the teeth, close the mouth, and perform kumbhaka. Lower the chin to the throat while you do this. After a count of about ten, exhale completely through the nose.

- Inhale through the teeth with a hissing sound
- Hold for ten seconds
- Exhale

No need to do this and sitali; one of them is sufficient. Same as with sitali, practice this especially when hot, or emotionally unbalanced. It is also a great practice for anytime there is inflammation, including asthma.

One-to-Two Breathing—Relax and Repair

Scientists as well as yogis have studied this breathing technique of one-to-two breathing. They found that when the exhalations are longer than the inhalations, the parasympathetic system is activated, which activates the immune system and calms the nervous system. It also induces muscular relaxation and is very effective in stress management. Some women find this to be helpful during menopausal hot flashes.

It is very easy to practice this breathing technique, and even ten rounds can make a huge difference. You can use it anytime you need to slow down, become calm, relax, or fall asleep. Yes, this actually helps a lot with insomnia. When you have trouble sleeping, you can practice this in bed on your back for ten rounds, and then roll onto your right side for better sleep.

Method of practice: This can be done sitting or lying down on your back. If on your back, you can have a blanket rolled under your knees for comfort. Breathe in through both nostrils at the same time for a count of four and then out for a count of eight. Note that any length of breath is fine as long as you keep the ratio 1:2 (2:4. 4:8, 8:16 etc.).

- Inhale fully for a count of four
- Exhale slowly for a count of eight

Though at first pranayama *may* be challenging, and many times, we feel that breathing is less important than the physical yoga poses, please do not underestimate these practices, and give them the time they deserve. These pranayama and breathing practices are a wonderful bridge into meditation. Practice them individually or as preparation for either your asana practice, or for meditation. They are the oxygen and energetic food for your body and soul.

— 6 —

Food and Nutrition

Food and nutrition affect our lives on many levels. Beyond the obvious weight loss, or control of weight, eating the right foods in the right manner will also have enormous effects on our yoga poses, pranayama, and meditation; prevent disease and illness; and improve body functions on all levels—from eyesight, hair, and nails, to better skin, liver function, and overall health and longevity.

Eating healthy will help you gain better joint movement, increase flexibility, and improve muscle tone, and thus improve your yoga poses practice. Food affects our mind as well. Clean food helps us maintain mental clarity, a steady mind, and emotional balance.

The opposite is also true. Drinking alcohol, eating heavy foods, or consuming too much dairy or animal products, may cause us to feel more stiff in our body, have a harder time breathing in pranayama, *and* feel more sluggish and less focused in meditation. The four elements of the flexitarian (yoga poses, pranayama/breath work, meditation, and food and nutrition) support each other, and food is one key element that really affects all others dramatically.

Listen to your body! This is true for anything physical we do, and it applies to food and nutrition as well. We all have different bodies, different levels of stress, different activity levels, and different prior conditioning. If foods that are recommended here or elsewhere do not work for you, there is no need to eat them. However, it is important to distinguish between emotional and physical reasons for avoiding certain foods. Emotional avoidance should be looked at, solved, and moved through.

While some food intolerances will resolve on their own once the diet is in balance and overall health is achieved, it is important to listen to your body and not eat foods that do not agree with you.

Eating in the Yoga Lifestyle Way

Eating healthy many times means eating more at home or cooking more, shopping for better ingredients, and saying no to certain foods and drinks we may have been used to consuming. The first step is to understand what is good for us. Then we actually try and incorporate this knowledge as much as possible into our yoga lifestyle.

The most important shift in our consumption of food is to make vegetables your priority. Vegetables contain phytochemicals, which are powerful health boosters. Vegetables will also help your body become more alkaline. Most people eat far more acidic foods (animal products, sugar, processed foods, white flour, etc.) than alkalizing foods (most fruits and vegetables, sea vegetables, Asian mushrooms, etc.). Aging is directly associated with acidity in the body. Note that flavor is not a good indicator for whether a food is acidic or alkalizing. For example, lemons, while they may taste acidic, are actually alkalizing in the body. Increase both the quantity and the variety of the vegetables you eat; have a rainbow of colors on your plate, but especially dark leafy greens. If you do nothing other than increase your dark leafy green intake to at least five ounces a day and decrease your sugar to a minimal amount, you will be taking a powerful step in the right direction.

Eat fruit as well, but try and always consume it between meals as a snack or as a stand-alone breakfast. Fruit digests quickly in the body, and thus needs to have clear passage through our digestive system, otherwise it may get stuck behind heavier foods and begin to ferment (not in a good way).

Have different textures on your plate and use a variety of cooking techniques. Bake, steam, ferment, and stir-fry, but try to avoid deep-frying. Eat three meals a day as well as healthy snacks for continued energy. For snacks, think of fruits and nuts, carrots with tahini, nori sheets, or a green smoothie. Eat at least one food item raw or live with every meal. This can be a small salad or a vegetable. The uncooked vegetable has living enzymes that will help with digestion.

The Quality of Your Food

Return to nature. Eating food that looks closest to its form in nature is always best. Processed or packaged foods often go through some sort of processing that decreases the nutritional value of the food and usually diminishes the taste as well. Canned tomatoes and pumpkins (in BPA-free cans) are an exception. Frozen foods maintain most of their nutritional value, though some may lose vitamins such as C and B when they are blanched before freezing to eliminate the enzymes that degrade the food.

Make it a habit to read food labels. If there are too many ingredients or many that you do not recognize, try switching to a different product. Seek organic, local, and fresh food. Eating organic simply means eating the way nature intended food to be—the way the world ate for centuries. Organic guarantees your food does not have enormous amounts of pesticides, hormones, or antibiotics, as well as tastes better and supports more traditional ways of farming that are sustainable to the planet. Another important element of buying organic food is the assurance that your food is not genetically modified (GMO). Genetically modified foods have been made to resist pesticides as well as grow better with specific chemical fertilizers, so it is better to avoid GMO foods.

How to Identify Organic Foods

With so many varying label standards, it can be tricky to know what you're looking for until you're used to it and it becomes second nature. Here's a tip: Look for a "9"on the product's sticker. Single-ingredient food, such as an apple or banana, should have a little sticker with a product number. If it is organic, it will begin with a 9. On a package of a single-item food, such as milk or chicken, you may find the USDA symbol of certified organic on the package. In packages that contain a variety of ingredients, such as ready-made food, processed foods, or beverages, there are different "levels" of organic. Here are terms to watch for:

- *100% organic:* This means all ingredients are organic and you may find the USDA organic seal.

- *Organic:* These products contain at least 95 percent organic ingredients (by weight). The rest of the ingredients are not available as organic. You may still find the USDA organic seal.

- *Made with organic ingredients*: These items must contain at least 70 percent organic ingredients. You will not find the USDA organic seal on these products. You may see something such as "made with organic quinoa, millet, and rice." (Up to three organic ingredients can be shown on the front of the packaging.)

If the product has fewer than 70 percent organic ingredients, those ingredients may be listed as organic only on the information panel. You will not find the USDA organic seal on these products. Since the use of the USDA organic label is voluntary and is costly, you may find smaller farmers that grow organic produce without any certifications or labels.

Choose Whole Foods

Most animals consume their food whole. Horses don't spit out the apple seeds. Okay, we are not horses, but there is a reason for nature being the way it is. When you eat a whole egg, you get both the protein of the white part as well as many other nutrients in the yolk, which are not in the white. When you eat a whole carrot, you get the nutrients, the sweetness and the fiber. When you drink just the juice, you get most of the nutrients, and since most fiber is removed, you get more concentrated fruit sugar. That is not the worst thing, but it can surely throw you off; when the fiber is removed, the juice causes the sugar levels in our blood to rise faster.

I make exceptions and have a juice or eat tamari (soy sauce) or miso. Save less edible parts of your vegetables and animal products—such as parsley and broccoli stems, leek greens, and bones—for stocks and broths.

Most whole foods contain more fiber and thus release the sugars in them slower (lower on the glycemic index), thus giving us long-lasting energy without the sugar crash.

Apart from vegetables and fruit, consume grain in moderation: all varieties of rice, quinoa, oats, millet, spelt, buckwheat, and barley are good options.

Try and reduce or eliminate wheat products, especially if you have gluten intolerance. Try going gluten-free for two weeks and see how you feel. If there is a dramatic difference for the better, then consider going completely gluten-free. Notice, though, that some gluten-free flour mixes have many things in them—some not so great. If you do go gluten-free, consider reducing or eliminating flour altogether.

Everyone would benefit from eating fruit instead of a muffin, a smoothie instead of processed cereal, and quinoa or rice instead of bread.

Drink Water

Our bodies are made of 70 percent water. Water nourishes as well as detoxifies. It contains amazing energy and is said to help bring harmony to our bodies. Drink eight to ten eight-ounce glasses of purified or spring water a day, depending on what you eat and what you do. If you are eating lots of soups and juicy fruits, you might need less water, and if you are sweating because of exercise or because it's just very hot out, drink more. A good way to keep in check is by observing your urine. Light straw color is what you want. If it is completely clear, you might be drinking too much (not good either!), and if it is dark, you need to go get a drink of water.

Start every day with an eight-ounce glass of water with juice from half a lemon (or whole if you can take it). This will both cleanse and replenish your body after the night. It will also get your bodily fluids moving.

Water is involved in nearly every bodily process, including digestion, absorption, circulation, and excretion, and helps carry toxins out of the body. When feeling tired or sluggish, drink two glasses of water, to improve circulation and alertness. It can be a substitute for a snack. Drink your water in between meals so you do not dilute the digestion acids in the stomach while eating. Drink your water at room temperature to match your body temperature, and in the winter drink slightly warm water, to keep your body warm.

Sugar

Ideally, eliminate sugar. It weakens the immune system and promotes aging and yeast overgrowth. It hurts your eyesight, promotes candida, increases cholesterol, rots your teeth, and makes you fat. Sugar, as well as high-fructose corn syrup, contains fructose, which goes to the liver, where it is converted to fat that contains the bad kind of cholesterol. Sugar has no positive nutritional value and is addictive. You get the picture?

Food and drinks around us are loaded with sugar and its alternatives. A can of soda has eight teaspoons of sugar in it. Most cereals are loaded with sugars. Sugar is added to most processed food—even bread, tomato sauce, ketchup, protein bars, milk substitutes, and most diet products—so it is hard to avoid it. Eat whole foods, home cooked or from sources you trust.

Read labels! Sugar comes in many forms and names. Here are just a few: cane sugar, corn syrup, fructose, honey, sucrose, maltodextrin, dextrose, molasses, brown rice syrup, white grape juice, maple syrup, date sugar, beet sugar, succanat, and lactose. Maple crystals, maple syrup grade B, honey, and date sugar are better for you than the rest as they are less processed and contain some additional nutrition benefits.

I have now switched to eating raw desserts (for snacks) or snacks that contain fruit, and so I no longer use sweeteners. In most recipes, you could probably use less than a quarter of the amount of sweetener suggested and still have it be plenty sweet. If you crave a sweet treat, try the bliss balls recipe (in the recipe section of this book), eat a piece of fruit, half a teaspoon of honey, or a chocolate smoothie of blended avocado, bananas, and cocoa (see www.doronyoga .com for more.)

On the bright side, with less sugar in your diet you will most likely be overall healthier with more consistent energy. You will suffer from fewer colds and less sickness, have healthier teeth, fewer cravings, and lose some weight or have an easier time keeping your weight steady. You may notice dramatically improved skin that will also age less. Less sugar means better mental stability and fewer mood swings. In the long run, you will have an overall happier feeling.

Sugar cravings can be emotional or physical. For emotional cravings, you will need to find the source and work on it until you make peace with it and it no longer triggers the reaction of eating sugar. The need for dessert can come from habit or the perceived need to balance something you ate. As for physical cravings, they mostly come because something else in the diet is missing—usually fat or protein. Healthy fats include avocado, olive oil, walnuts, coconut oil, flax seed, hemp, chia seeds, sesame seeds, nuts and nut butters. It is better to eat whole-fat products such as whole milk or yogurt than low-fat or fat-free products because the substitute for fat in low fat products is usually sugar.

If you do decide to eat a less healthy dessert (such as ice cream), serve it on a separate plate. Add healthy toppings, such as berries, nuts, or cacao nibs so you need less of the sugary dessert. Take a moment before you eat to appreciate the food. Then take a bite and keep the food in your mouth. Feel it there—the flavor, the temperature, and the texture. Slowly let it melt and, only then, swallow. This is meditation in action.

A better option is to take a moment before you get your dessert in the first place. Maybe start with just a bowl of fruit. Take grapes or berries or a peach, and eat slowly—the same way as you would the dessert. Many times, if five minutes have passed since the initial moment of craving, the craving has actually disappeared.

Coffee and Caffeine

Coffee can provide some benefits, such as increased energy and a sense of alertness, both of which are temporary, but caffeinated coffee has many downsides as well, so it's best to reduce it to a minimum. Caffeine can cause mood swings, dehydration (it is a diuretic), acidity in the stomach and mouth, and some even say, joint stiffness. Some other problems with coffee are not necessarily about the coffee itself. Many drink their coffee with sweeteners and dairy, which are not great for you.

Try green tea instead of coffee. Green tea is high in antioxidants and contains much lower levels of caffeine. There are also grain coffees that can be good replacements. Herbal teas are my favorite; they are fun and healthy. You can drink mint tea after lunch for digestion, chamomile at night to calm down, rooibos tea with a hint of non-dairy milk for breakfast, or licorice tea for taste and to aid with breathing. You can also try a cinnamon stick with mint or ginger, or one of my favorites drinks—fresh lemon ginger with a hint of honey.

Dairy

The best dairy is mother's milk for infants. If you are not an infant any more, consider consumption of dairy to be a luxury. Dairy can be nurturing and even emotionally healing, though it can also cause mucus and phlegm, let alone suffering for the animals that produce it.

The most common sources of dairy are from the milk of cows, goats, and sheep. Our bodies are more similar to those of goats or sheep, and thus it is easier to digest these smaller animals' milk. If you have any inflammation, breathing issues, mucus, or bloating, it is wise to avoid dairy all together. If you are consuming dairy for protein or calcium, you can find better ways to get both. For example, tahini is wonderful for both calcium and protein.

When choosing cow's milk, look for organic, grass-fed, and, if available, raw or at least non-homogenized (cream on top). Homogenization is the process of forcefully straining the milk so that the fat is broken down. This is done so that when we open the bottle of milk, we do not find any cream on top. To get your food minimally processed, use non-homogenized milk and simply shake the bottle for a moment before pouring the milk out. It's that simple.

Raw milk or raw unpasteurized cheese contains healthy bacteria and enzymes. It contains lactose and lactase. Lactose is the sugar, and lactase is the enzyme that likes to eat the sugar, and so it actually digests the lactose for us. Most people have an easier time digesting raw milk as the lactose is predigested. Even people with lactose intolerance may tolerate raw milk better.

Yogurt with live cultures or kefir (fermented milk) are dairy product that are easier to digest than most other dairy products. They are high in protein and contain healthy bacteria for your gut. If you have to keep one dairy product in your diet make it yogurt or kefir, although non-dairy versions of these products are also available, such as coconut water kefir. Try to drink milk substitutes instead, but watch for additives that may have negative influence on your health. You might find the best option is to create your dairy alternatives yourself. Coconut, almond, oat, or hemp milk are good substitutes and making them from scratch is actually quite easy!

Should You Be a Vegetarian?

The quick answer is YES. Even better yet, be a vegan and eat mostly raw food. But this does not work for all of us, all of the time. Being vegan does not automatically mean being healthy. Many vegan items are highly processed, unnatural, or contain GMO. Some of us do not digest beans or certain nuts, and will have a harder time being vegan. Some of us will simply crave animal product and feel better with small amounts of them in our diet.

The blood type diet for example, suggests that beyond the basic ability of most people to eat vegetables and fruit, people with blood type A have the easiest time being vegan. Many of them will not crave meat or dairy. People with blood type B have the best ability to digest dairy, thus are more prone to being vegetarians (true for people with blood type AB as well). People with blood type O, the most ancient blood heritage, are better off eating a hunter-gatherer's diet, mostly vegetables with limited amounts of animals.

I tried exploring this on myself as well as researching it with dozens of my friends and students. My brother is blood type A, and does not crave meat, can digest hummus and beans in general, and is better off with no dairy. I, on the other hand, am blood type O, cannot digest beans (even if sprouted, fermented, cooked with seaweed, etc.) and really crave meat once in a while. I do not do well with dairy. This is what led me to become a flexitarian. Morally and ethically, I wanted so badly to be a vegan. I really do not want to harm anything or anyone. I tried, but did not feel well. What worked best for me was dramatically increasing the amounts of vegetables, nuts, fruit, and quinoa in my diet and also adding small amounts of fish and chicken, just a few times a week.

I am not recommending you eat meat just because you are blood type O, but rather really check and see. What happens when you reduce meat? How much can you eliminate and still feel good, or even better? Whatever blood type you may be, the basic rule always applies: Eat lots of dark leafy greens! Vegetables and fruit are the foundation and main ingredients of any healthy diet.

Fish, Meat, Poultry, and Eggs

If you decided to eat animal products, do it with awareness and gratitude, a basic principle for consuming animals. Fish is your best choice, preferably smaller oily fish (wild when possible) as these are low in saturated fat, high in protein, contain omega 3, contain less heavy metals, are usually less processed than meat, and easier to digest.

Poultry is high in protein, contains B12, and is easier to digest than red meat. Eggs provide a whole range of nutrition benefits, from protein to vitamins and minerals. Make sure to buy good quality, free range, organic chicken and eggs.

Two main things that are extremely important about eating meat are the quantity and the quality. Eat small portions. You don't need much meat to get the protein or the vitamin B-12 fix. Avoid processed meats, such as salami, ham, or any other cold cuts, unless you find brands without nitrates.

Note that many meat cravings can be solved by simply using the same seasonings you may use for your meat on non-meat options such as tempeh or in nut pâtés.

Inspiring Diets

There are a few diets that inspire my way of being. I do not follow any one of them 100 percent all the time, but rather take the best from each of them and adjust my diet with some of their wisdom in mind.

Macrobiotic Diet

The macrobiotic diet recommends a great deal of brown rice. It also recommends a large amount of vegetables alongside the rice, as long as they are not from the nightshade family (potatoes, tomatoes, eggplant, peppers, and chilies). Spinach and Swiss chard are not nightshades but may affect us the same way.

Nightshades contain an alkaloid called solanine, which is a compound that contains small levels of toxicity. The nightshade family plants have this compound in order to ensure their survival. It is more prevalent in plants that have been picked before they are ripe. When the plant is ripe (and the seeds are ready to be spread), the level of toxicity is reduced greatly.

For many people, eating a variety of plants including the nightshade family will not be harmful, especially if they are organic local plants that have been picked ripe (or grown in your backyard). For some, green peppers will be worse than red or orange peppers (as they are less ripe when picked), and for some, eggplants or tomatoes may be just fine, especially if seeds and skin are removed. The bitter taste of some of these plants is the protection mechanism, so try to get the least bitter forms. You can always observe and see how you feel after eating them. Listen to your body; it will tell you what to eat and what to avoid.

Those on a macrobiotic diet do consume fish but not meat or dairy. When I tried this diet for a while, I felt great. I found that it was especially nourishing for me when the season turned colder—in fall and winter. The diet includes many hardy root vegetables, brown rice, tempeh, soups, and stews. It also includes fermented foods, which help with digestion. Today, I still incorporate most of the macrobiotic food concepts with added raw foods and a bit less grain.

Review of Macrobiotics

Eat brown rice and fermented foods. Eat plenty of cooked vegetables of a variety of colors, but eliminate nightshades. Eliminate dairy and meat, but eat small amounts of fish.

Raw Food Diet

Eating raw food is wonderful and important. There is a difference, though, between eating some raw food, and being completely on a raw food diet. Eating only raw food has many benefits and can be used as a temporary cleanse, especially in the summer. The powerful enzymes in raw foods stay alive, thus bringing great energy into the body.

This being said, it also increases vata, and for those with vata imbalances—those that find their mind is wavering or those that have a hard time staying grounded—raw foods may not be the best choices, because they will only increase the feeling of lightness. Furthermore, trying to adhere to a raw food diet in the winter when the weather is cold may not be what your body asks for. Raw food diets may recommend heating your raw soups lightly (to under 115–118 degrees, depending on the diet) to get the warmth without killing the enzymes.

Eating raw food is an excellent way to balance a meal. Add a raw salad or fermented vegetables as a side dish or cut up some carrots, radishes, or kohlrabi and place it on the side of your plate.

If you eat your salad as a main dish, just add some protein (cooked or not) and fat to it. Your protein may be nuts, beans, sardines, or some grilled chicken. Most of the proteins contain fat already, but you can also add olive oil and avocado to get some healthy oils in. The fat helps us feel satisfied and full.

More ways to increase raw food in your diet are by eating a smoothie a day and eating raw food as snacks. You can have a raw smoothie for breakfast as a pick-me-up to start your day or between your lunch and dinner. Keep raw foods readily available. I always have fresh, seasonal fruit on my counter ready to eat, or sprouted beans or seeds in the fridge. Place some carrot sticks in a jar with water, and whenever you feel like a snack, it's right there ready for you. I share the recipe of my bliss balls, which is my main afternoon snack, in the recipe section.

Another snack I love is soaked almonds. I place the almonds in a small bowl with water in the morning, and in the afternoon, I have almonds that have begun their sprouting process. They are now alive and easier to digest. Use raw almonds for soaking. You may find raw dehydrated almonds in the store. This means they were soaked, and then dehydrated at low temperatures to keep the enzymes alive. These days you can also find a variety of raw snacks in health food stores. My favorites are kale chips and raw chocolate.

There are many people today that claim that the raw food diet helped them overcome illnesses and increase energy. You will need to explore this for your body and see how you feel. I definitely recommend increasing the amount of raw food, especially fermented foods, in your diet.

Note that the Ayurvedic diet generally does not recommend uncooked food, claiming that it is hard for your body to digest it. For this reason, it is best to add raw food in moderation according to what your body is able to digest. As a flexitarian that appreciates both the Ayurvedic principles as well as the raw diet principles, I try to find balance: more raw food when it is warm outside or when I am feeling sluggish, and more cooked food when I feel ungrounded and scattered or if it's cold outside.

How to incorporate raw food into your diet
- Eat some raw food with every meal.
- Eat raw foods as pick-me-up snacks.
- Eat more raw food (especially fruit) when the weather is hot and humid.
- Eat more raw fermented food in the winter.
- Make one meal a day mostly raw food.
- Add raw smoothies to your meal plan.

Ayurvedic Diet
Using the system of Ayurveda as a platform to build and maintain a healthy diet is an excellent part of living a holistic life. Ayurveda—the science of life—has general recommendations for a healthy diet, as well as specific ones for each dosha. Though I do not follow the

Ayurvedic diet to its exact recommendations, there are many things about it that are worth following as you have already seen in the Ayurveda section. I especially appreciate Ayurveda's recommendations for harmonious and holistic eating.

In some of main ways, my diet differs from one based on Ayurvedic principles, including incorporating more raw foods, especially when blended. At times the Ayurvedic diet recommends dairy (especially to balance pitta), yet I recommend reducing it to a minimum.

Your diet will likely change from day to day depending on the season or geographical area you are in, as well as the circumstances in your life (job, relationships, hormone fluctuations) and your mental state of being. Eat a diet that will either bring you into balance based on your specific body constitution (your individual ratio of vata, pitta, and kapha) or one that will maintain your balance. Many of us, when out of balance, tend to be imbalanced in vata, causing us to be less focused, productive, and grounded.

Ayurveda is a holistic system and takes into account the food, the eater, and the process of eating. The food is looked at on many levels. What does it taste like? Is it of high quality and where does it come from? What are the effects of this food on the doshas? Does it have any medicinal properties?

The eater in regard to food is mostly the digestive system and all its components. How well is the digestive system functioning? If there are problems, are they physical or emotional?

As for the process of food, Ayurveda recommends taking a moment of silence before the meal and maybe offering gratitude to the food and the process it took for it to arrive to us. Ayurveda advises to chew the food slowly and thoroughly.

Ayurveda describes six tastes: sweet, sour, salty, bitter, astringent, and pungent. Each one has different effects on us when we eat it in excess, as well as specific effects on each dosha.

A well-balanced Ayurvedic meal includes all six tastes, unless you are trying to balance a specific dosha.

- A vata balancing diet will favor sweet, sour, salty, hot, heavy, and oily.
- A pitta balancing diet will favor sweet, bitter, astringent, cold, heavy, and oily.
- A kapha balancing diet will favor bitter, astringent, pungent, hot, light, and dry.

The Six Tastes According to Ayurveda

1. **Sweet:** rice, grains, fruit, milk, oils, nuts, fish, meat. Promotes growth of bodily tissues; an emollient that increases strength and soothes the senses. When eaten in excess, effects are: obesity, lethargy, dullness, mucus, breathing issues, coughing. Sweet food decreases vata and pitta and increases kapha.

2. **Sour:** lemon, cheese, yogurt, sour fruits, fermented foods. Promotes digestion and salivation; improves flavor. When eaten in excess, effects are: thirst and deterioration of muscles and teeth. Sour food decreases vata and increases pitta and kapha.

3. **Salty:** salt, sea vegetables. Promotes digestion and cleansing; a laxative that enhances flavors. When eaten in excess, effects are: thirst, skin problems, too much acidity. Salty food decreases vata and increases pitta and kapha.

4. **Bitter:** leafy greens including radicchio and endive. Cleanses the palate; improves skin condition and digestion; anti-inflammatory and anti-bacterial; removes fat and helps detoxify the blood and body. When eaten in excess, effects are: deteriorates tissue, reduces strength. Bitter food increases vata and decreases pitta and kapha.

5. **Astringent:** vegetables, legumes, autumn fruit. Promotes healing of wounds; promotes fluid absorption; sedative. When eaten in excess, effects are: drying of tissue, constipation, loss of vitality, gas retention. Astringent food increases vata and decreases pitta and kapha.

6. **Pungent:** spices, herbs. Improves body functions; detoxifies; improves digestion; sharpens the senses; purifies the blood; promotes circulation; stimulating. When eaten in excess, effects are: weakened virility, fatigue. Pungent food increases vata and pitta and decreases kapha.

SOME AYURVEDIC EATING PRINCIPLES

Start with clearing out foods that are not good for you. This includes leftovers. Eat freshly cooked meals, ideally meals made with love—maybe you even cook them yourself. Eat the right amount, not too much, but also not too little.

How you eat matters. Eat slowly and in a calm manner; eating when stressed is like ingesting poison, so sit down to eat, take a few breaths before your meal to calm, and maybe even feel some gratitude.

What you eat matters. Eat sattvic foods—foods that are organic, holistic, easy to digest, and rich in flavor. These foods will promote a calm and focused state of being. Avoid tamasic foods and toxic ingredients—food prepared using plastic, aluminum, and non-stick cookware made of Teflon; foods cooked in a microwave; foods that have been processed and/or refined, and preservatives, artificial flavors, and artificial colors; these will increase negativity, pessimism, ignorance, laziness, and doubt.

Sip warm water throughout the day to allow food to flow easily. Eat in harmony with nature, in a clear state of mind and with care and love. Eat fresh and consume just the right amount. Enjoy, as food is a gift.

AYURVEDIC DIET BASICS FOR YOUR DOSHA TYPE

Vata has a tendency to be too light, floating, and distracted. Eat warm and cooked foods to ground and steady vata. Avoid excessive consumption of raw fruits and vegetables as well as very cold foods such as ice, ice cream, and frozen foods.

For breakfast, aim for some grounding food, especially when cold. Consider oatmeal or polenta. For lunch, try adding some lightly sautéed kale to your rice or quinoa. For dinner, try a simple baked salmon with some warm grain and cooked veggies. Squash is a great vegetable for vata people in the winter. To all your meals add healthy fats such as walnuts and avocados. Use warming spices such as cardamom, cinnamon, clove, cumin, and ginger, but avoid very spicy or bitter foods.

Sip warm water or non-caffeinated herbal teas to keep moist. Most importantly, stay calm and grounded. A bowl of brown rice with some avocado is a fantastic recipe to get grounded.

Pitta has plenty of fire in it, so eat cooling foods such as smoothies with lots of greens and/or fruit. Choose spices that are not too heating, such as turmeric, cinnamon, fennel, mint, and thyme. Eat sweet, seasonal fruit such as pears, apples, watermelon, berries, etc.

Eat them separately from your meals, or as meal substitutes. Eat more carrots, leafy greens, asparagus, and broccoli as well as grains such as basmati brown rice or barley.

Ayurveda does recommend the use of dairy to balance pitta, particularly warm milk and honey before bed. I use coconut milk or almond milk instead. Eat more sweet and bitter such as rice, fruit, and a bit of honey or maple. Reduce salty, spicy, and pungent foods, especially vinegars; they may cause heart burns. Keep it light, cooling and naturally sweet to keep your fire working but not burning.

Kapha enjoys a diet that is lively and full of energy to awaken the fire within, and reduce heaviness. Aim for foods that are light and dry, with a bitter or pungent taste, and avoid foods that are sweet or salty. Eat some raw food with all your meals to help spark the digestive and metabolic systems. Choose lighter foods such a fresh vegetables and avoid oily foods, especially fried food. Eat only small amounts of nuts and seeds. Include fruits such as apples, pears, and pomegranates in your diet, and make sure to have your meals regularly. Do not skip meals.

When needed, use honey as a sweetener and stay away from all other sugar. Ginger tea is good for stimulating the digestion. Enjoy it with or after meals. Remember, light and alive food is the food of choice for kapha.

The most important thing for all doshas is to keep a calm and clear mind. Do your best without stressing about it. Choose a combination of dosha foods that you like and that will bring a smile to your face so that you enjoy eating. Let the entire act of eating be a joyful experience within a nice environment where you can eat consciously and slowly, giving yourself plenty of time to digest.

Distinguish Between Physical Hunger and Emotional Hunger

Practicing awareness is always important but not always easy. My weakness is nighttime when I am alone. Sometimes I think that food will fill a perceived emptiness by creating a feeling of love and connection. During these times, I notice that I start looking through the cabinets and fridge for some comfort food. It is not always easy to stop while this is happening, so the next morning, I sit for a few moments and relive the night before in my mind. As I envision myself opening the fridge, I imagine myself stopping and checking to see if I am feeling physical hunger or emotional hunger. Then I imagine recognizing that it is emotional hunger and I close the fridge and smile to myself for a moment while finding gratitude for something good in my life. I take a deep breath and then go to floss and brush my teeth.

You will need to recognize when it is that you have a weakness and go to food as comfort. Once you recognize when it happens, you will need to sit and envision a new pattern of behavior—not during the event itself, but when you are calm and in control. After you envision a new way of behaving, you then need to practice it during those times of weakness. Over time, you will simply notice this entire process in a split second, before it actually happens, and you will be able to skip the emotional eating.

Since for me this happens at night, I have also made sure to eat enough earlier on so that it does not become a physical hunger blended with emotional hunger, which can lead to the worst binging possible.

How to Deal with Emotional Hunger

It all starts with awareness. Recognize when your weak moments are, when do you go for food not because you are hungry? Learn to be present and know the difference between physical and emotional hunger.

Empower yourself by reconditioning your mind when you are strong, not when you are in a weak moment. Envision yourself acting as you would like to at a different time than when you're actually losing control. Practice this kind of mindfulness regularly as it normally takes a month to make or break a habit or recondition your mind. Most importantly, don't give up. It will change! Just stay with the practice.

Harmonious Eating

How you eat your food is almost as important as what you eat. For example, you may eat great organic food in front of your computer while stressing over a problem you have—this will convert the great energy of the food into negative energy. There are a few rules that will help you receive the maximum benefit of the food you eat.

Principles of Harmonious Eating

Check your hunger level before eating and eat until you are close to full but not completely full. Always eat sitting down in a relaxed manner; better not to eat when you are emotionally upset. Eat food that is as fresh as possible—real food—not processed food.

Warm your food to at least room temperature and serve it on a plate. Do not eat out of the pot. Chew well! Gandhi said, "Drink your food and eat your water." But have water after your meal, or take only small amounts of warm liquid during the meal. Eat your main meal before 3:00 pm, and give yourself time between meals to digest. Give yourself a few minutes after you eat to rest or take a slow walk.

Eat what you enjoy and enjoy what you eat!

Creating Your Menu

Unless you are good with your eating habits, in order to make sure you implement the new changes you want, you must create a menu for the week. It is not an easy thing to implement the suggestions in this chapter. They sound reasonable, but when actual life kicks in, there is always a reason to slip.

As a flexitarian, we of course allow some flexibility, but as someone working on becoming a flexitarian, it is most important that you begin with a bit more of a rigid diet, and once you can stay with it, allow for more flexibility. This is not to say that you need to beat yourself up for slipping, but you do need to have the intention to stay with it, at least for one month.

Most people have great difficulty implementing these suggestions unless they sit down once a week (at a time when they are well-rested, fresh, and relaxed) and plan every meal for the week ahead.

Tips to Help You Manifest Your New Eating Habits

Make a meal plan for the week according to the season and your needs. Shop over the weekend for at least the first half of the week. Ideally cook fresh for every meal, but realistically you may want to cook some basics over the weekend so you have staples ready to go for the week. You can make your lunch the night before.

Make your fruit/nut/seaweed/healthy snack visible to you either in the fridge or on the countertop and have some form of fruit or vegetable washed, ready to eat, and sitting in front of where you work. Have ingredients for your green smoothie ready, so when hungry you can always make one easily.

Plan your dinner before you leave the house in the morning and have the ingredients ready to go in the morning or pick them up on your way back home. Stick to your plan, even when it is tempting to stop for pizza instead. Have ten handy recipes that you like and can easily make, and try to memorize them, so that cooking becomes easy.

Distinguish between physical hunger and emotional hunger and use your yoga and breathing practices to maintain emotional well-being.

Healthy Snack Alternatives

I love grazing. Between my meals, I get a bit hungry, and want a little something to keep me calm and steady. This may be because I am mostly pitta, but in case you also like to eat between meals, it is good to be prepared with the right snacks. If you do not have healthy snacks ready, you may be tempted by less healthy ones, which I hope you no longer keep at home.

Here are some healthy options.

- Chopped vegetables
- A green smoothie
- A banana chocolate smoothie (see recipe)
- Carrots with tahini dip or on their own
- Celery with almond butter
- Nuts (best: walnuts, Brazil nuts, and almonds; also fine: cashews, pecans, and hazelnuts)
- Seeds: pumpkin and sunflower (preferably raw and sprouted)
- Nori sheets (the dry roasted seaweed sheets that are used for sushi)
- Fruit
- Small amounts of dried fruit, preferably with no sulfites especially if you are allergic to them or have asthma
- Slice of bread (or better, veggies) with hummus or tahini

Last Meal of the Day

For most of us the last meal is dinner. Ideally you would have it at 5:00 pm, brush your teeth, and not eat any more until you go to bed at 10:00 pm. Then you would eat breakfast after your morning practice at 8:00 am or 9:00 am, so you would actually get to do a fast—or cleanse—every day. For most of us, this will not work. Pitta types, especially, may need to eat some extra calories before bed. However, do try to have your last meal at least three hours before bed.

I do recognize that we are all different, and some will really need a small amount of food later, hopefully a small snack and not a burger or even a big handful of nuts. Not eating two hours before sleep allows the food to digest so that the body can rest while sleeping and not waste energy on digestion, which at times influences the mind (i.e., dreams) as well.

I know that if I eat chocolate at night, I tend to have much crazier dreams. If possible, eat your last meal earlier, as this allows for a longer time for your body to rejuvenate. Remember, if there are ten to twelve hours between the time you eat at night and your breakfast, it is like having a daily fast; it helps keep your colon clean.

Foods for Maintaining a Healthy Body

Some foods work better for us humans, though we still may have different needs. The food I recommend here will help keep your body healthy. The easiest to remember is vegetables. Simply eat more of them, in all colors, and especially dark leafy greens, like kale, collards, bok choi, mustard greens, arugula, and baby salad mix (antioxidant nutrients, fiber). You can also make raw vegetable smoothies or juices to increase vegetable consumption and thus increase the intake of good vitamins and minerals.

Sprouts contain live enzymes and vitamins, and are great with food or as a snack. Seaweed is a great source for minerals, protein, and fiber. Try to add them to your diet at least a few times a week, and even daily. Pineapple, turmeric, and garlic have good anti-inflammatory properties and help the body heal from inflammation internally. You can add them to your food, smoothies, and teas (turmeric with lemon and honey).

Be creative, and change things around, but have some staples that you do not give up on, such a smoothies, green salads, or your 4:00 p.m. apple and two Brazil nuts snack.

Recipes

These are some of my basic favorites that I use often. Of course you will eat a greater variety of meals than what I offer here, but it's a good jumpstart for some healthy, easy to make recipes.

Meals and Snacks

BREAKFAST SMOOTHIES

When it is not too cold out, I love having a smoothie after my practice or simply fruit. If the morning is cold and I feel like eggs and avocado, then I'll have my smoothie as my 4:00

p.m. pick-me-up snack. Since anything can go into a smoothie, you are welcome to play and experiment. My foundations always include some greens (dark green or red lettuce, baby kale, bok choi, collard greens, celery), some fresh herbs (parsley, cilantro, mint) juice from a whole lemon, ½ inch of ginger, and seasonal fruit. The fruit I use the most is apples—an apple a day makes my smoothie sweet and happy. If kiwi is around, then I would add one or two kiwis to the smoothie, mango when in season, grapes in the summer for extra sweetness, banana if I want it thicker and silkier, and berries and other fruits according to season and availability.

Even with a very strong blender you will need to add water, juice, or ice. I like water, and at times a small amount of pomegranate or apple juice. Try not to be tempted to make it too sweet. Keep a nice amount of greens and limit the juice. You can add to this any superfood powder, for extra vitamins, minerals, healthy fats (omega 3), or protein. Most of these you can use regularly, but use them in small amounts, switch them around, and take some breaks. I like spirulina (an algae that contains vitamins, omega 3, and protein), hemp seed (also omega 3 and protein), chia seeds (protein, fiber, omega 3), or maca (energy, sexual function, and sweetness).

My Classic Green Smoothie

Ingredients

- 5–8 oz. baby kale or baby salad mix

- 1 apple

- 1 kiwi

- 1 cup pineapple (fresh or frozen)

- 2 tablespoons lemon juice (more or less the juice of 1 lemon)

- ½ cup water (or as much as you need to get your blender moving)

- ½ teaspoon spirulina

Procedure

Begin with pulsing the blender until you have all the ingredients blended some, and then slowly increase the speed. Let it run a minute or so on the highest speed to get a smoother consistency. Drink your smoothie immediately. If needed save some for later, but try and drink it the same day, as nutrients disappear as it sits.

Almond Milk

Ingredients

- 1 cup raw almonds, soaked in water
- 4 cups filtered water
- 2 medjool dates, soaked, or honey, or maple syrup (optional)
- vanilla bean (optional)
- ¼ teaspoon cinnamon
- pinch of sea salt

Procedure

Soak the almonds overnight or for eight hours with ¼ teaspoon sea salt. This will help them come to life and break down the phytic acid and enzyme inhibitors in the almonds. If you have less time, a couple of hours will do, but it is much healthier to soak for longer. Drain the almonds, rinse them, and place them in a blender with the water. Blend on high for three minutes till smooth and creamy.

Drain through a cheesecloth or use a nut milk bag. Squeeze the bag well to get all the liquid out. Return the liquid to the blender, add cinnamon (and optional dates and vanilla bean), and blend for another minute or two.

Store in a glass jar for three to four days.

Quinoa

Here's to one of my favorite foods that just so happens to be good looking, great tasting, and flexible, as well as healthy. It works amazingly in everyday cooking, as well as in fancy meals. Quinoa, "the mother grain," the "gold of the Aztecs," has been a staple food of the Aztecs for thousands of years, and since the 1980s has been cultivated within the United States. Quinoa is one of the most complete foods in nature. It contains all nine essential amino acids, enzymes, vitamins and minerals, fiber, antioxidants (manganese and copper), and phytonutrients.

Quinoa is an incredibly healthy replacement for grains (it is gluten-free) and an excellent source of protein (it is highly recommended for vegetarians). Add quinoa to your superfoods list along with kale, garlic, hemp, and blueberries. It is great for regulating blood pressure and preventing certain diseases, and overall, it strengthens the entire body. It is easy to cook and can be enjoyed all year round.

Easily digestible, you can add quinoa to your favorite warm winter soups or to a refreshing summer salad. The seed is related to the spinach and beet family; it is light, fluffy, and slightly crunchy with a delicate and subtly nutty flavor. Quinoa flour can be used in cookie and muffin recipes, and noodles made from quinoa make delicious pasta.

Quinoa is coated with a toxic chemical called saponine, so it is important to rinse it well before cooking. As with most food, consume quinoa in moderation. A few times a week is enough.

How to buy: When buying quinoa, make sure there is no moisture in the packaging (or bin if buying in bulk). Store quinoa in an airtight container. It can last for several months, especially if placed in the fridge. When deciding how much to buy, remember that quinoa expands to several times its original size once cooked.

How to cook: Soak quinoa for a couple of hours before cooking (optional). Make sure to thoroughly wash the quinoa (removing the saponine) by placing it in a meshed strainer, running cold water over it, and rubbing the seeds between your fingers.

Basic Quinoa Recipe

Ingredients

- 1 cup dried red or white quinoa
- 1¾ cups organic vegetable broth
- 1 teaspoon salt (optional)

Procedure

Rinse dried quinoa in a strainer or strain soaked quinoa and rinse. Place in a medium-size pot and dry-roast for three to four minutes, until nutty smell appears. Add vegetable broth, cover, and bring to a boil. Lower the heat and cook for fifteen minutes, until liquid is completely absorbed. Turn off the heat but let the covered pot sit on the burner for another ten minutes before serving. When cooked, the grain becomes translucent with a little white half-moon (the germ), making it very pretty.

More Quinoa Cooking Ideas

Quinoa salad: Add your favorite chopped veggies to the quinoa as soon you turn off the heat. They will warm up, as the quinoa sits for ten minutes. Try substituting quinoa for couscous in a Moroccan feast or use it instead of pasta in your pasta salad recipe. Add quinoa to your tomato soup or stew.

Curried quinoa and peas for simple and quick lunch: Add frozen peas, garlic, ginger, and curry (or just turmeric) to your quinoa to make a delightful presentation. Quinoa is also good cold in salads. Combine chilled quinoa with pumpkin seeds, diced carrots, adzuki beans, cumin, cilantro, salt, and scallions. As an option, add a bit of lemon juice.

Did you think of quinoa for breakfast? Make a delicious breakfast cereal with quinoa, fruits, nuts, cinnamon, and maple syrup (grade B).

Explore! Quinoa is very versatile.

A note of safety: Quinoa contains moderate to large amounts of oxalate. Individuals with a history of calcium oxalate-containing kidney stones should limit their consumption of this food.

ENLIGHTENED KALE

Kale is super healthy, but not always enticing. I find that eating it warm with additional fat and flavor makes it a delight. In the recipe below, you can substitute a bit of tamari (wheat-free soy sauce) or even just salt and pepper for the nutritional yeast.

Ingredients

- 10 oz. kale (about one bunch), stems removed, rinsed and chopped. Save stems for stock.
- 1 tablespoon coconut oil
- 1 cup organic stock (I use organic free-range chicken stock, but veggie stock is great too.)
- ½ cup nutritional yeast

Procedure

Heat oil in a deep sauté pan. Add stock and kale and cook for approximately five minutes. Remove from heat and add nutritional yeast (sprinkle liberally to taste).

Variation: Cook the kale only in stock and then add 1 tablespoon of olive oil and the nutritional yeast. Add a dash of salt if desired.

Baked Zucchini

Here is a very quick and easy recipe that goes well as a snack or as a side dish to almost anything. Most people love it, as it is simple. If you do not like cumin, simply bake the zucchini with salt and pepper and maybe a bit of sweet paprika.

Ingredients

- 4–5 medium zucchinis
- 3 tablespoons olive oil
- 5 cloves of garlic, thinly sliced
- cumin seeds (or powder)
- salt to taste

Procedure

Preheat oven to 350 degrees.

Wash and cut the zucchini lengthwise into about ¼-inch slices, but really don't go measuring. I normally cut them either in half or thirds. Place zucchini in a bowl and mix with oil. Transfer zucchini onto a baking sheet. I use a silicon sheet, but you can use any baking sheet. Sprinkle cumin, garlic slices, and just a bit of salt over the zucchini.

Bake until it begins to turn golden. At times, I bake it very little as I like it crunchy, but many prefer it softer. If you prefer it softer, check every ten minutes with a fork to see if it is soft enough. Explore; you can't go wrong. You can even eat it raw.

Salmon Asian Style

Most of us are lacking in our essential fatty acids (EFAs), essential nutrients that we need in our diet. They help our brain functioning, nervous system, hormones, and blood circulation and will promote healthy skin. Salmon is an excellent source of EFAs. Other foods that have EFAs include walnuts, chia seeds, and flax seeds. However, even though I eat mostly vegetarian, my body and mind feel incredible if I eat fish one to two times a week. The body absorbs fish EFAs best. Below is a very simple recipe that tastes delicious and takes only about fifteen minutes, including preparation and cleanup. Ideally buy fresh salmon, or if you buy frozen salmon, defrost it in the fridge for sixteen to twenty-four hours.

Ingredients

- 2 scallions

- 2 tablespoons coconut oil

- 2 pieces wild salmon (4 oz. each)

- 2 large garlic cloves, minced

- ¼ cup mirin (rice vinegar—see note below for substitute)

- 2 tablespoons tamari (soy sauce)

- 2 tablespoons maple syrup grade B

Procedure

Thinly slice the scallions and separate the white from the green. Combine garlic, mirin, tamari, and maple syrup in a medium-size bowl to make sauce.

Heat coconut oil in a pan over medium heat and sauté the white part of the scallions in the pan over medium heat for one minute.

Add the salmon with the skin side down. Let it cook for about two minutes. You will see the salmon bottom starting to turn opaque. Pour sauce over the salmon and flip it over. Cook for another two minutes or so according to your taste. I like to leave the center somewhat raw. Garnish with the green scallions and enjoy!

Note: If you do not have mirin, you can use apple cider vinegar with a teaspoon of honey (*mix well*) instead.

SALADS

Playtime! Use lots of mixed greens as your base. To that I add avocado when in season and walnuts. Any veggie goes: carrots, radishes, sprouts, cucumber, etc. For fun, add nuts, seeds, olives, and at times a bit of dried fruit or goat cheese.

Kale Salad

Ingredients

- 5 oz. baby kale (or regular kale stems removed and then shredded to bite size)

- 2 tablespoons pumpkin seeds (toasted or raw)

- 1 tablespoon sunflower seeds

Dressing Ingredients

- 1 part olive oil

- 1 part lemon juice

- 1 part nama shoyu (or any other good quality organic soy sauce, including Braggs). Nama shoyu is unpasteurized and raw, so better flavor and more health benefits.

Procedure

Whisk all dressing ingredients well. Pour the dressing onto the kale and massage the dressing into the leaves until they are completely coated (and look bright green). The longer the kale sits with the dressing on it, the softer it gets, so sometimes I make it a few hours ahead. It also means that it will still be great the next day.

Kale Chips

Kale chips are a great healthy and yummy snack. They have a crunch to them, and satisfy that savory need, while providing the power of dark greens.

Ingredients

- 1 bunch kale*, washed, dried, and stems removed, or 5 oz. baby kale

For the marinade:

- 4 tablespoons tamari (soy sauce)

- 4 tablespoons nutritional yeast

- 4 tablespoons fresh lemon juice

- 3 tablespoons raw tahini

- 2 tablespoons water if needed to make tahini more liquid

Procedure

Mix all of the marinade ingredients until smooth and fairly thick.

Put kale in a large bowl (this may be done in batches), pour some of the marinade over the kale, and gently massage to coat all the leaves.

Arrange kale on dehydrator sheets being careful not to overlap.

Dehydrate at 125 degrees for about two hours until crisp. It is possible to do this in the oven at the lowest heat setting available.

*Bunches of kale vary so when I need to increase the volume I continue to add equal parts of the ingredients.

Condiments

SALAD DRESSINGS

Keep it simple! The classic Israeli dressing is to mix two parts olive oil with one part lemon juice, and a bit of good quality salt. That's it. Switch the lemon juice with orange juice and orange slices for fun. You can add some mustard and capers for diversity. Add a bit of curry and honey for an Asian feel.

Tahini Dip/Sauce

Tahini can be eaten as-is from the jar, but I love the dip/sauce as it is flavorful, satisfying, rich in calcium, and a fantastic dip! Dip carrots, cucumber, blanched broccoli, cauliflower, whole-wheat pita bread, or crackers. You can also eat this with rice, diluted as a sauce for falafel, or as a thick dressing on salads.

Ingredients

- 4 large garlic cloves
- 1 bunch parsley
- 16 oz. organic tahini
- 8 oz. water
- ⅔ cup lemon juice
- salt to taste

Procedure

Peel garlic cloves and place in food processor. Pulse a few times or until garlic is finely minced. Wash parsley. Cut off the very end of the stems (about one inch) and discard. Cut the rest of the stems from the leaves and place in food processor. Pulse until finely chopped. Add the leaves and pulse until finely chopped.

Add the tahini. After emptying the tahini container, fill half of it with water, close the container with the lid, shake well, and then pour the water into the food processor. Pulse until all ingredients are mixed well.

Add lemon juice and salt. Pulse and taste. If needed, add more salt. If it is very thick, add a little more water as it will thicken even more once it is in the fridge. Pulse until ingredients are evenly combined. Place in covered glass container in the fridge. Tahini will last one week in the fridge.

Zchug

Zchug is one of my favorite foods from home. Very common in Israel, brought by the people of Yemen, it is known as the "hot stuff," and the traditional recipe is far too spicy for me. I created my own variation with emphasis on the cilantro, giving it spice with garlic. Zchug is very popular as a condiment for falafel. I also eat it with bread, rice, and raw veggies. Enjoy zchug anytime, but it is especially great during the spring and summer for a nice cleanse. The cilantro, garlic, olive oil, and lemon juice are excellent detoxifiers.

Ingredients

- 3 cloves garlic
- 1 medium-size bunch cilantro
- 2 teaspoons fresh-squeezed lemon juice
- 2 tablespoons extra virgin olive oil
- ½ teaspoon salt (taste and add as needed)

Procedure

Rinse the cilantro well and cut off the ends of the stems to use them for stock. Spin the cilantro in a salad spinner until the cilantro is dry. In a food processor, add the ingredients separately in the following order: garlic, cilantro, lemon juice, olive oil, and salt. Mix well after each ingredient is added. Store in a glass container and eat within five days of preparing.

Pesto

Traditional pesto is made with basil, pine nuts, and Parmesan cheese. I took the liberty of playing around and created this variation. Try it out and feel free to keep exploring on your own. Remember, it is always great to learn from tradition, but never be afraid to step out of it. How about mint walnut pesto?

Parsley Almond Pesto

The parsley almond pesto tastes amazing with pasta. I love to have it with brown rice pasta, but I would recommend trying it with any of your favorite pastas. It is so good, that sometimes I just put it on a slice of bread and enjoy. Maybe make it into a sandwich and add some lettuce, tomato, or anything else you enjoy (a roasted portobello mushroom, for example).

Ingredients

- 4 cloves garlic, minced
- 1 very large bunch parsley
- 1 cup olive oil
- ¾ cup almonds
- sea salt

Procedure

Place garlic in a food processor and pulse until finely minced. Add parsley and pulse until finely chopped. Add almonds and run the food processor while slowly adding the olive oil. Add salt. Start with a pinch, pulse a couple of times, taste, and add more salt if desired.

Sweet Recipes
Bliss Balls

This is the perfect pick-me-up snack that will take care of your sweet tooth. It is healthy, delicious, and gluten-free. If you are like me and need seconds, make the bliss balls smaller. When I do not have much time to make these, I make them without the chocolate coating, as that is the most time-consuming part.

Ingredients

- 1 cup pitted dates
- 1 cup dried apricots
- ½ cup raw almonds

- ½ cup raw Brazil nuts
- ½ cup raw walnuts
- ¼ cup raw pumpkin seeds
- ½ cup raw sunflower seeds
- ¼ cup goji berries
- 2 tablespoons chia seeds
- 3 tablespoons whole sesame seeds
- 2 tablespoons tahini
- 7 oz. dark chocolate (72% cocoa or above)

Procedure

In a large bowl, mix the above ingredients except for the dark chocolate thoroughly. Place half of the mixed ingredients in a food processor. Pulse until the mixture seems sticky. The ingredients do not need to become completely smooth, but just of a good consistency to roll into a ball. You may see that the dates, apricots, Brazil nuts, and walnuts are blended, but some sunflower seeds, goji berries, and pumpkin seeds are still whole. With your hands, make small balls, and place them aside.

Place the rest of the mixed ingredients in the food processor, procees, and again with your hands, make small balls and place them aside.

Melt the chocolate in a double boiler (if you do not have a double boiler, fill a medium-size pot with two cups of water and place a slightly smaller pot on top with the chocolate inside; do not let the water from below boil over into the smaller pot or the chocolate will become chunky and difficult to spread). Keep the temperature on low and continue to mix until the chocolate is completely melted, then take the pot(s) off the heat. Wait one minute (no longer) for the chocolate to cool.

With a spatula, place a spoonful of chocolate on top of each ball and use your fingers to spread it over the ball, and then place it on a plate. I cover around half to three-quarters of the ball so that it does not stick to the plate. Place the bliss balls in the refrigerator. They should be ready to eat after an hour. Store them in the refrigerator and eat within two weeks.

CHOCOLATE MOUSSE

Ingredients

- 2 large ripe bananas

- 1 ripe avocado

- 3 dates (or more if you like it sweet)

- 3 tablespoons raw cocoa powder

- ½ teaspoon maca powder (optional)

- 1 tablespoon cinnamon

- 2 tablespoons cacao nibs (optional—for a bit more chocolate crunch!)

- 1+1 cups almond or coconut milk

- Raspberries or strawberries for garnish, optional pecans or goji berries

Procedure

Place all ingredients apart from one cup milk in a strong blender and begin blending. Pulse at first, and then let the blender run for two to three minutes. Add as much of the second cup of milk as needed to make the blender move and to reach the consistency of your choice.

Note: This dish is beautiful with some pecans on top, adding a nice crunch, raspberries or strawberries in season, or goji berries anytime. Sometimes I even add five chopped strawberries into the mousse after it is blended.

Supplements

Supplements are like insurance. Do not rely on them to give you the nutrients that you need. Though there are many studies that show the benefits of taking supplements, there are also concerns about the long-term effects of using them regularly. So remember—first have an awesome healthy diet, then supplement just as much as necessary for specific needs.

Since I add the superfoods spirulina, hemp seeds, maca, and chia seeds to my diet regularly, I do not need to supplement as much. I take my multivitamin on days that I do not have a large green smoothie. I take my omega 3 fish oil once in a while when I feel I did not get enough fatty fish, chia, or spirulina. I take vitamin C if I am feeling that my immune system is not as strong as usual.

Below you will find some general guidelines for supplements. Since many multivitamins really do not contain high enough levels of actual vitamins, it is important to seek out a good brand. Look for vitamins that come from natural sources and whole foods rather than chemicals, and again, rely on a wholesome diet. Supplements are your safety net.

Please meet with a nutrition consultant to find what is right for your specific needs. These are just general guidelines, and many of us will not need to follow all of these recommendations. Take only what you need.

Multivitamins

The amounts are a range of what is safely recommended. I added in parentheses the preferred amount that you may find in stores.

- Vitamin A (retinol): 5000 IU
- Vitamin A (from beta carotene): 5000–25,000 IU (10,000 IU)
- Vitamin C: 500–1000 mg. If you take vitamin C separately, it is not crucial to have it in your multivitamin.
- Vitamin E: 100–800 IU (400 IU)
- Vitamin D: 100–400 IU (400 IU)

B vitamins

- B1 (thiamin): 10–100 mg (50 mg)
- B2 (riboflavin): 10–50 mg (50 mg)
- B3 (niacin): 10–100 mg (50 mg)
- B6 (pyridoxine): 25–100 mg (50 mg)
- Folic acid: 300–600 mcg (400 mcg)
- B12: 10–50 mg (50 mg)
- Biotin: 100–300 mcg (100 mcg)
- Choline: 10–100 mg (50 mg)
- Inositol: 10–100 mg (50 mg)

If it is difficult to find a multivitamin that has enough of these B vitamins, you can take a separate B complex supplement.

Minerals

- Boron: 1–6 mg (2 mg)
- Calcium: 250–1250 mg (1000 mg)
- Chromium: 200–400 mcg (300 mcg)
- Copper: 1–2 mg (2 mg)
- Iodine: 50–150 mcg (150 mcg)
- Iron: 15–30 mg for women; men do not need this
- Magnesium: 50–400 mg (250 mg)
- Manganese: 10–15 mg (10 mg)
- Potassium: 200–500 mg (not a must)
- Selenium: 100–200 mcg (100 mcg)
- Zinc: 15–45 mg (15–20 mg)

Boron, magnesium, calcium, and other minerals are important, yet many multivitamins do not contain amounts even close to the daily recommendation of these nutrients. Because of that, a mineral complex may be advised as well, unless you eat sea vegetables (seaweed). Consult with your nutrition advisor.

You may also find other ingredients in your supplements such as ginseng, garlic oil, and many other herbs that can be beneficial.

- Omega 3: 1000 mg with meals

How to Eat Healthy Without Spending Much

I keep hearing that eating healthy is for the rich—that organic is too expensive—and that fast food is cheap. This may seem true on the surface, but look at the bigger picture. Eating well will allow you to stay healthy and clear-minded. It reduces the number of sick days and medications you will need and keeps you joyful so you have a better life now and a longer, healthier life down the road.

Today organic food is so prevalent that at times it costs about the same as or even less than non-organic (especially when you buy it in season). I've purchased organic olives for much less than the non-organic. You just need to be a wise shopper and learn where to find good prices.

Tips on Buying Healthy for Less

Buy fruits and vegetables that are in season, when they're at their best. Usually there is an abundance of seasonal options that are fresh and cost less. Summer offers blueberries, cherries, broccoli, asparagus, beets, and watermelon. Fall offers apples and pumpkins. Spring is a joy of greens, sprouts, and apricots, and winter offers root vegetables, kale, and more. Of course, this depends on where you live.

Buy locally to save on shipping costs and help preserve a healthy environment.

Eat only what you need to. Serve yourself on a small plate. Go back for seconds if needed. Don't be tempted to eat from the pan or the package. Reduce the cost of food by reducing waste.

Buy whole foods like whole grains and vegetables. Raw ingredients can make great simple meals, while processed food is less healthy and can be more costly.

Use the whole food. Use stems in smoothies or for stocks. Eat all parts of the broccoli. (You can shave the outer edge of the broccoli stem and then cut it into strips to use with dips or just as a snack.) Eat the radish and beet leaves, and buy small fish like sardines so you eat the whole fish.

Cook at home. When I compare the seemingly high price of organic chicken (or any other food item I buy for home cooking) with a regular meal out, I realize that using the best ingredients at home is still far less expensive than a mediocre meal out.

Fresh and Healthy—How to Choose the Freshest Fruit and Veggies

If your food looks great, fresh and appetizing and is organic, the produce is probably good. Knowing the source is always a plus. Growing your own is ideal, but for most of us this is not going to happen.

Tips for Choosing Fresh Fruits and Vegetables

Buy local. Locally produced food does not need to be transported, so there is a better chance it was picked ripe, has less waxing and coatings, and less energy was wasted in bringing it to you. Check the sticker on the fruit to see where it's from.

Buy organic. Get food that is grown the real way, the way nature planned it. The sticker on fruits and vegetables will have a number. If it starts with a 9, you're good to go.

Go to a farmers' market. Get produce directly from the source.

Buy in season. Ideally ripe fruit directly from the farmer or that is locally grown, so it is more likely to have been ripened on the tree. Fruit that has been ripened on the tree tastes better and has more nutrients.

Some Ways to Check Ripeness

Touch gently. Most fruit and vegetables should be firm but not too hard.

Take a look. Fruit and vegetables should appear vibrant and appetizing with no signs of discoloration or mold.

Tap on a watermelon with your hand. A deep hollow sound is an indication of ripeness and sweetness.

Take a look again. Greens, specifically, should look vibrant and alive; if they have started to yellow or wilt, move on.

Check the bottom of the garlic to see if it looks clean or if some black mold has started to grow.

Smell. Most ripe fruit should smell good.

Smell again. Onions should have no odor.

Touch again. Cantaloupes should be slightly soft to the touch and smell like cantaloupe.

Pluck a leaf. Pineapples are best when a leaf up top is easily plucked out and the bottom of the fruit smells like pineapple.

— 7 —

Mind Work

By now you may already be practicing yoga and pranayama regularly, eating better, and starting your day with an intention. Isn't this enough? Indeed taking care of your physical body is important and helpful, but it is not enough. Our health—physical, emotional, and spiritual—is affected a great deal by our mind, and without training the mind, we may find that health and happiness are still not guaranteed. The Buddha said the mind is everything; what you think, you become.

Why Train Your Mind?

My dad ate healthy and was in pretty good physical shape, but his mind was in constant worry and stress. He was bothered by why there were greedy people in his workplace and worried about whether my mom still loved him. He worried about us—his kids—and always expected more than what was realistic. He did have a heart condition as a child that may have remained minor throughout his life, but his state of mind affected his state of physical health, and he suffered a great deal because of this until his early death, at the age of sixty-four, from a heart condition that led to a stroke. True, doctors had not diagnosed him with stress—this is my observation. I have seen this over and over with students of mine, as well as with myself. The only times I get sick are when I enter my worried state of mind.

The good news is that with a sound, clear, and healthy mind, we have the ability to support our body as we eat better and exercise. We even have the ability to transform the feeling of unhappiness that can arise while we are ill or when life is not as we would hope for it to be.

Challenges are unavoidable. Life contains good and bad, ups and downs. We will always be exposed to the spectrum of life, no matter how well we take care of ourselves. There are many unpredictable things that can happen at any given moment. To experience the full gamut of life and not fall into suffering, we must train our minds to be disciplined, to not react in auto-mode and to not add stories and unnecessary value to a situation.

We can improve our immune system with the power of our mind and with our breath. Our mind, our willpower, and our determination are powerful healing tools.

Swami Vivekenanda said, "Whatever you think, that you will be. If you think yourself weak, weak you will be; if you think of yourself strong, strong you will be." Your mind is very powerful, and your thoughts may actually change your reality. By training the mind, we become its master; we consciously create the reality that is good for us, and thus are capable of remaining happy beyond the circumstances that life may throw our way.

Taming the Beast: The Art of Focusing

Meditation is the intention to train the mind. We train the mind so that we can see reality for what it is, so that we are able to live our lives not through the projections or stories made up by our minds but through the direct experience of life.

Meditation can be practiced sitting on a cushion in what you may imagine as a classic Buddha picture, with eyes closed or half closed, finding bliss. And it can also be practiced throughout your life in everything you do. You will learn different techniques for meditation so that in different situations you can choose the one most appropriate for you. You may gravitate towards one more than the other, and that is completely fine. We train our bodies with yoga poses and our breath with pranayama practices. Our mind needs training as well. For many of us, the mind is the master and thinks at will and sometimes even causes us to speak and act in manners that our true selves would not choose.

The training of the mind goes through stages. The first is focusing, learning to keep the mind steady, even if not still. Focusing the mind will eventually allow the mind to drop away completely and not interfere with the true perception of reality. When seeing reality for what it is, you may come to experience higher states of realization—different levels of consciousness.

The practice of focusing the mind is done either by withdrawing from our perceptual senses (seeing, hearing, smelling, etc.) or by focusing the mind with one sense on one object, such as eyes on a candle or ears tuned in to a specific sound or music. We slowly become the masters of our mind. Think of a bicycle. When we get off the bicycle, our legs do not keep moving in the same manner as when we were pedaling. Our feet stand firmly on the ground, keeping us steady. As part of the process, we will train the mind to work and be active when it is needed and to be at rest when no thinking is of use. Focusing on one point allows the mind to slow down, thus creating a feeling of calmness and space, which are beautiful side effects to the training process.

Meditation takes an intention, not an effort. With no intention, nothing will happen; however, meditation needs to be effortless.

Tips to Help You Train Your Mind to Focus

- Practice doing one thing at a time.
- Gaze at one object and stay with it for a while.
- See with your eyes, and notice the mind stepping in to give interpretations.
- Practice allowing the interpretations to float away. Stay with the object.
- Think only when you need to. (Don't expect to succeed right away.)
- Stay with what you are doing until you are done.
- Create an environment with fewer distractions.

Setting Up Your Space

It is helpful if you can set up a small place that will be your regular meditation area. It can even be a corner of your living room with something symbolic to represent something good, calm, and peaceful. Some people like to place a little statue of a Buddha to remind them that they are practicing, realizing their own Buddha nature (enlightenment). Maybe for you it is a flower, a crystal, or any other small object that allows you to feel safe, in peace, and calm. It may be a collection of objects. These are not things that you worship but rather mood setters and gentle reminders of your purpose, reminders to drop away from your habitual mind, from whatever was happening in your life before you came to look at this little altar.

The only thing you really need for meditation is a cushion to sit on. You can have it in your meditation space regularly, or if there is no room, you can tuck it away and pull it out every time you sit. There are plenty of dedicated meditation cushions out there, but anything that will elevate your seat and be firm enough to help you keep a tall spine will do. If the cushion is placed on a carpet, wonderful; otherwise, consider placing a folded blanket underneath your ankles or knees, depending on your sitting style. Your sitting area should feel very welcoming. It should be a place that you want to go to, a place of refuge, a safe place where you feel comfortable dropping away your worrying mind and just being.

Review of Setting Up Your Space

Set a dedicated space for your practice. Create a small altar; it can be just a flower or a candle. Have a cushion or other object to sit on (bench, chair) and keep the area clean and welcoming.

Meditation: Zen Basics

Zazen is the fundamental practice of Zen. It is the practice of sitting in meditation. When looking at a group of meditators in a Zen monastery, you may think that everyone looks similar, sitting tall and still with eyes lowered, but it is what is happening in the mind that matters. Zazen meditation is a process. The simple instruction is *just sit!* For most of us this is not an easy task, and just sitting is neither fun nor easy on the mind. Zazen uses the tool of the breath to begin the process of training the mind.

Meditation Instruction (Zazen Meditation)

Sit as in the breathing exercise. Lower and soften your gaze in front of you. Keep your eyes open or half open. Drop your awareness inward and observe your breath in the belly area.

Begin with counting the breath to help you stay focused. Count each inhalation and each exhalation. As you inhale, count one, and as you exhale, count two. Count to ten, and then go back to one. If you lose your count, just go back to one. Let thoughts come and go while you keep returning to your breath. It is sometimes shocking to see how hard it is to count to two without drifting away. Don't give up. Smile every time you lose the count and come back to one. It is only with practice that it gets easier, so just stay with it. Before you know it, it will become very soothing.

We all have different "break out" times, the moment where the mind yells "enough!" Many times, the mind has a great excuse. There is an e-mail that needs to be written just this second, or maybe you just have to drink some water and then you will come back. Normally, when we give in to the mind's demands, we reinforce its control over us. It is when we sit through these moments of distraction that the training of the mind begins taking place.

Start with five minutes, and increase your sitting time by one minute every day until you reach twenty or thirty minutes and sustain that. If you find it easy and accessible to sit longer, wonderful. Go for it.

REVIEW OF ZAZEN MEDITATION PRACTICE

Sit in a comfortable position with your spine tall. Lower your eyes and tune in to your breath at the belly. Count your breath—inhale one, exhale two. Count to ten, and then start over again. If you lose your count, simply go back to one.

Start with five minutes and increase the time daily until you get to twenty or thirty minutes. Use a timer, so you do not need to worry about the time.

Sky Meditation: Soft Focus, Clear Mind

Sitting in zazen meditation is a great way to begin training your mind. It will help you gain focus and steady your mind. After doing zazen for many years, I discovered that I needed to soften and try less. This is where the sky meditation came in. Sky meditation is a meditation of surrendering—of allowing.

Sky Meditation Instructions

Sit quietly and be an observer. Do not try to resolve anything. Listen to your breath, and observe the thoughts that pass by. You will be like the empty sky accepting any cloud coming by, noticing, but not holding on to any cloud. The sky does not choose the clouds; it does not hold on to them or control them. Try to be like the sky, notice your thoughts, but let them keep moving. Do not add any stories, remarks, labels, or preferences.

Observe your thoughts and your body. Who is it that is observing? Are you your thoughts? What happens when you just let the thought float away without cultivating it?

Try to set a timeframe of at least twenty minutes. It takes some time to be able to drop into the place of sky. There is no limit to how many times you can do this. Get up after twenty minutes, stretch your legs, smile, and go back to sitting. If there is no time (and somehow there never is), dedicate time once or twice later that day to sit for another twenty to thirty minutes. It really helps to do this often, as then you will notice which thoughts are constantly coming up. You will start seeing patterns, and answers will start being clear without you even needing to look for them.

Review of Sky Meditation Practice

Sit in a comfortable position with your spine tall. Close your eyes and become an observer. Let go of what you observe. Notice what comes up next. Let go of what you observe.

Visualization: Object Meditation

Object meditation is similar to Zen meditation, but with this meditation, you keep your awareness and attention on an external object, either one that you can actually see or an image within your mind.

This meditation is particularly helpful as a tool for staying in a meditative state while functioning in the "real world," since you will learn to be able to keep your mind focused and calm on everyday objects.

Object Meditation Instructions

Sit comfortably with a tall spine, and set your gaze softly on an object in front of you, hopefully something you find pleasing. Take a deep breath.

Options may include the flame of a candle set three to four feet away from you, a flower, or even a tree. When gazing at the object, find a balance between focusing on the object and finding softness with the gaze so that you are not seeing any one specific detail.

It is important that as you gaze at the object, you are not tempted to use words to label what you are seeing (do not use adjectives such as green, tall, small, beautiful, dying, etc.). As you gaze at the tree, you are simply seeing the tree for what it is with no interpretation or labeling from the mind; do not go inward and drift into thoughts or stories about the tree, and try not to allow what you see to remind you of other trees in other situations, thus bringing in stories from your past or creating fantasies about the future (the tree house from childhood or the swing you want to hang on it, for example).

This meditation is not easy at first as the mind is very well trained to see something and immediately associate it with a word. Sometimes I call this meditation "the art of non-labeling." If labeling or stories come in, remember not to be hard on yourself but to simply take action and just return to the simple activity of only seeing.

The beauty of this meditation is that it can be practiced anywhere, anytime. You may be waiting for a friend outside a café and while you are waiting, you practice looking at a tree, a flower, or even a knob on a door. Maybe you have a favorite tree that is right outside your window or balcony, and gazing at it regularly helps you discover the tree from a completely new perspective.

I used to take breaks from creating my art to sit on my small balcony and stare at a huge tree that was pretty much blocking my whole view. I would sit and simply lose myself in the tree. I would look with some distracting thoughts at first, and then the more I surrendered into just seeing the tree, the more the tree revealed itself and became much more beautiful than I have ever seen it before.

REVIEW OF OBJECT MEDITATION PRACTICE

Sit in a comfortable position with your spine tall. Find something pleasing to stare at and simply look blankly at the object and let yourself surrender into it. As thoughts come in, allow them to float away and return to simply seeing your object.

Imaginary Object Meditation Instructions

Bring into your mind an object or being that you find very pleasing or that you feel unconditional love towards. It may be your favorite animal, flower, or person. See it clearly within your mind's eye. Begin noticing every part of the object. If it is an animal, for example, begin with the head. Observe the eyes, the nose and ears, the fur, and the entire face; take your time to really get to know what you are envisioning. Keep going through the entire body if this is your vision, or simply remain with the head. You want to eventually see it as clearly as if it were there in front of you, allowing it to fill up the whole concentration of the mind and all of its space.

Thoughts may appear, either about your object or something else. Simply return to your object over and over again. Over time, the image will become more and more familiar and associated with a good feeling of calmness and relaxation.

We learn that just by bringing the object to mind, the signals of centeredness, focus, love, ease, and so on will be "attached" to the image, and thus it will be easier to enter this state of mind. The mind will obey and release faster. When a distraction happens in life or the mind gets agitated, close the eyes for a moment and return to *the object* with a sense of allowing—letting *the object* be—without interruptions.

REVIEW OF IMAGINARY OBJECT MEDITATION PRACTICE

Sit in a comfortable position with your spine tall. Bring into mind the image of a pleasing object or being to focus on. Study your object without labeling it and get to know it. See the object in your mind's eye and keep "looking" at it. As thoughts come in, allow them to float away and return to simply seeing your object.

Mantra Meditation

Mantra meditation, or *japa*, is the practice of repeating a word, a name, or a sound over and over again. Normally, this word or sound is either given to a student by the teacher or has a special symbolic meaning to the student. Sounds and words that might work for you are a word or a name that represents something you look up to, or see as representative of goodness, wholeness, love, or enlightenment.

Since my mind already has the tendency to lean towards words, I prefer to use more abstract sounds, as they allow me to drop away more quickly. The sound "*Ohm*" is one such example. It creates a vibration in the body, thus helping me physically as well as mentally as I drop away and relax. It may even be a short phrase such as "*Sat Nam*," which represents the true nature of who we are, or "*Ohm-Mani-Padme-Hum*," which is a classic Tibetan prayer mantra said to contain all of dharma (teachings) within it.

Find something that you can enjoy repeating that will become second nature for you so that if at any time you find yourself distracted, you can just bring in the mantra and repeat it to yourself, whether you are sitting in meditation position or driving to work. When you repeat it over and over it becomes a refuge—a place to go back to find your peace. You may stay focused on the sound or the meaning, but eventually allow yourself to let go of the observing mind and simply let the mantra take over. You will feel as if you and the mantra have united. The mantra is yours, so keep it special and meaningful for you.

REVIEW OF MANTRA MEDITATION

Choose a word or sound that resonates with you, or one of the chants below. Practice repeating it over and over. Allow yourself to be lost in the sound.

Chants

Chanting is a way of meditation and setting intentions. For some, the meaning of the chant is very important; for others, like me, the act of repeating sounds is what makes chanting powerful. The repetition of words that are considered powerful helps, and by focusing on the sound as it happens, we can be more present and maybe even drop from the mind into the heart space.

I chose three mantras that originate from the Upanishads, which are Hindu sacred texts, whose meanings I like and that are chanted by millions around the world. No need to fear religion; they do not require you to believe in anything and do not interfere with any belief you may hold.

Aum/Ohm

Aum (or Ohm) is the primal sound, or word. We chant this mantra from the *Mandukya Upanishad* to connect to the universal vibration, the energy that connects us all together.

Peace Mantra

OM SAHANA VAVATU SAHANAU BHUNATTU

SAHA VIRYAM KARAWAVAHAI

TEJASVI NAVADI TAMASTU

MA VID VISHAVAHAI

OM SHANTI SHANTI SHANTI

Together may we be protected

Together may we be nourished

Together may we work with great energy

May our journey together be brilliant and effective

May there be no bad feelings between us

Peace, peace, peace

Prayer for Enlightenment

OM

ASATOMĀ SAD-GAMAYA

TAMASOMĀ JYOTHIR-GAMAYA

MRITHYORMĀ AMRITAM-GAMAYA

OM, SHĀNTI, SHĀNTI, SHĀNTIH

From ignorance lead me to truth

From darkness lead me to light

From death lead me to immortality

Let peace prevail everywhere

Walking Meditation

Walking meditation serves as a release for the body between two sessions of sitting, as well as a gateway for bringing meditation to your everyday life. Though walking meditation is done in a controlled environment and the walking does not serve to bring you to at any destination, it is the practice of your meditation in movement that creates the challenge and begins to bridge your seated meditation to your daily life activities.

Begin your walking meditation very slowly. Stand tall; bring your left hand into a fist right below your belly button and wrap your right hand around it. Keep your shoulders relaxed, your neck long and your head tilted slightly down so that you are seeing the space just in front of you with a soft gaze. Maintain connection with your breath and drop your awareness all the way to your feet.

Begin taking your first step. Go as slowly as you need to in order to really be able to notice all of your movements. Be aware of every little detail—from the lifting of the right heel to the releasing of the ball of the foot and the toes from the earth, from the movement of the foot just a bit forward in front of you to the landing of the heel and the touching of the balls of the feet and toes to the ground. Notice the slight weight shift as the left heel starts to lift up and the balls of the feet release from the earth—and another step is taken.

Allow the movement to happen with your awareness but practice the art of non-labeling described earlier. Simply walk. No need to describe what you are doing; no need to tell yourself that the floor is cold or warm. Just be with it—let the sensations be. It is difficult to walk and meditate. It's like learning a new skill. The walking meditation may be short—six to ten minutes—between sitting sessions, or as a meditation on its own for as long as you feel comfortable.

Over time, experiment with increasing the pace of your walking. You may notice that it is easier as you increase the pace, but at a normal or faster than normal rate, it is hard to remain present. This is great practice for training the mind to stay present even as things speed up, and in modern day life, it appears as though life is constantly moving faster.

Review of Walking Meditation

Stand tall with shoulders relaxed and eyes lowered. Place your left hand in a fist below your navel and wrap your right hand over it. Walk slowly with awareness of every movement. Increase the speed of your walk when you can maintain a steady mind during the slow walk.

Meditation in Everyday Life

Bliss is possible both on and off the cushion. Meditation is a fantastic tool, a wonderful school for unlearning, for training the mind to not be attached to the conditioning it has engrained within it. It is important that you begin your training in favorable conditions, in a quiet and supportive place.

You also have the ability within the practice of meditation to drop into places that would not be functional off the mat—levels of consciousness that are beyond the functioning of space and time where you can experience absolute bliss beyond your body and mind. Since a great part of your daily life does require your body to function and your mind to make decisions or execute tasks, you will need to learn how to take these tools of meditation and cultivate them while sitting so they can become useful in your daily life. This is where the practices of object meditation and walking meditation help build a bridge between meditation on the cushion and functioning in the real world. Begin to practice everything you do in life as a meditation.

You can begin with some simple tasks such as brushing your teeth. At first, you will need to move almost in slow motion so that you can really practice awareness of the fingers opening the cap of the toothpaste, pressing the thumb to squeeze the tube, seeing the toothpaste on your toothbrush without labeling it, and placing the toothbrush in your mouth. Be mindful of every movement, knowing exactly which part of your mouth has been cleaned already; be aware of the pressure, the taste and the texture of everything that is happening at the moment without using words to describe it.

Of course, just now, I have used words to explain the process, and thus words have an important role. Just remember to use them only when it is important for communication, while at other times be fully with the experience that is happening at the present moment.

Another such practice would be eating in meditation. You may notice new flavors, new sensations, and a lingering enjoyment of the process. When eating with awareness, you are no longer in auto-mode. There is an explosion of flavor with every bite. When you chew rice longer, you will discover its sweetness as it releases its natural sugars in the mouth.

Start with small practices of mindfulness in your life, especially routine ones like brushing the teeth or eating a meal—or even just a piece of fruit. Over time, allow these practices to expand into all parts of your life—opening your bag to reach for your keys, placing a glass of water back on the table, switching the light on, driving, and every other action you take in life.

Meditation is needed on and off the mat so that eventually your whole life is one big continuous meditation, an experience of the present moment in which you are mindful of all you do, leading to an existence of bliss at all times.

Review of Meditation in Everyday Life

Practice being aware of small tasks in your daily life, then try to do them without labeling the actions you observe. Start with simple awareness practices, such as mindfulness as you brush your teeth. When you eat, chew slowly and notice every flavor, smell, and texture. Use these practices with all of your activities in life.

Experiencing Life Here and Now

When we are fully present with the moment in front of us, the little mundane things appear magical and supreme. Have you ever watched raindrops make patterns of circles in a temporary asphalt pond? These moments are precious, and last just as long as you are fully there. The moment you wish you could share this with someone, is the moment it is gone.

You can practice being in the moment with specific actions. In Japan, drinking tea is an entire ceremony, one that is a practice of awareness in action. Try to make your own ceremony. Watch the stream of water as it flows into the kettle. Later, watch your hand as it lifts the kettle to pour the water into the teacup. Look at the tea first. Just observe; no need to describe what you see. Then smell it. Take a moment—no rush. Watch your hand as it lifts the cup to your lips. Take a sip. Let the liquid rest in your mouth for a moment. Experience the flavors. Take another sip and allow the warmth to spread through your body. No one else needs to understand this tea experience, and no one really can. The experience is gone, and what is left are words describing something that was not words.

Slowing down is a key aspect of being here and now, really seeing and experiencing the process. As you learn to see the little details, you also learn to see in slow motion the fast actions, such as riding a fast motorcycle.

Here is another example. I travel mostly on my own. Many times people would ask me, "Who do you tell to look at this wonder, or that amazing sunset? Don't you have a need to share what you are seeing? Is it even really amazing if you did not tell someone about it?" Some people travel to places that others have been to before so they can share the same experience. The trip to Paris, or the Venice canals. Others live their experiences through photographs. Some people are satisfied to just be able to tell their travel partner to look at something and then recall it later at dinner. Maybe they will add their own interpretation of the situation, or their own perspective of what they saw.

I have learned that the moment you speak of the wonder, the wonder is gone. It is no longer the experience but a story of the experience (which may be a wonderful experience on its own). It is never an easy task to portray an experience in words. Some gifted writers are capable of bringing experiences to life, but even then it is not the writers' experience, but rather your interpretation of what you are reading. Give five people the same story to read, and then ask them to draw or express what they have just read, and you will most likely have five new stories.

Let's get back to the trip. You are traveling with a friend and you really want him or her to see the sunset, or the castle, or the old woman on the street corner. What you may do, is call attention to what you want them to see, experience or enjoy, but don't describe the details. If the friend can divert the attention to it, and experience it without thoughts, they can find the same bliss and awe you experienced. The more detail you give, the more you put the friend at risk of focusing on your description and not the thing itself. The focus should be only on helping get the attention, and then allow them to enjoy what you saw. Trust that they are capable of seeing what you saw, and if not, it's okay.

The camera may be your good friend, as it is as close as possible to bringing the experience of what you saw to others. But in reality, it does not really show what you saw and experienced, but rather a fragment of it. It does not include your emotion, smells, weather, etc. Consider taking photos of what really moved you, even if is a detail of something, capturing a Zen moment rather than a common postcard.

When the experience is lived fully as a complete moment, it will be followed by many other amazing moments. Eventually, life becomes so full of these moments that there is nothing to lose, nothing to hold on to, just bathe in the presence of constant beauty.

There sure was a moment on my spiritual path, where life seemed lonelier than before. Most of the sweetest moments of seeing reality, as it truly is, the experience of bliss, are moments that cannot be spoken of. It is the knowing that others can experience this too, a deep connection with the universal energy, that allows the sweet understanding that the experience IS shared with others, just not through words.

There's Nothing Wrong with Thoughts

In many meditation classes you will hear: quiet the mind, stop thinking, calm yourself. But really, nothing is wrong with your thoughts; it's your attitude towards them that creates problems. Thoughts can come and go; are they yours? Are they you? When sitting, being aware, we notice thoughts come in. If all we do is notice and do nothing about them, they will go away. They have no reason to stay unless you hold on to them and encourage them. Thoughts are like clouds in the sky, they come and go, but does the sky care? Does the sky get irritated about them?

Be like the sky. Allow the clouds to be, and they will soon drift away. Try and fight them and they will persist. The peace of mind is within you and beyond you. There is no attaining peace of mind; there is allowing it to be there. You already have peace; it is just tainted by your thoughts, by your attitude towards them. When you let the thoughts fool you to believe that they themselves are who you are, when they create an identity that you hold on to—when you become your thinking—you lose yourself.

And the self you lose, is not the self you THINK you are. You lose your true self, the self that is beyond a momentary thought. The sky is not the sky that appears when clouds are there. That is just a sky with clouds. But the real sky is just sky. Like you, when you find the surrender, when you become a complete observer, when the thoughts pass through you without leaving a trace, then you realize yourself, you become the clear sky.

The Pain of Pain!

Imagine this: After your visit to the dentist, the bottom left side of your mouth was filled with sensation, unpleasant sensation. A sensation that caused discomfort, so much so, that you just had to tell everyone about it. Then you tried to do some work, but instead, you were constantly telling your colleague how impossible it is to work like this, how this dentist did a horrible job, how upset you are because you think that he did the injection wrong. This may not be a real scenario, but not an unlikely one. The frustration, the complaining and suffering can go on and on for a while, creating more irritation, and constantly making the situation worse. It is adding suffering to the pain that already exists.

Instead of being so upset with the pain and situation, you may recognize the sensation, and then let it be and move on to whatever else you need to do. Maybe your awareness is not as quick and you already labeled this sensation as "discomfort." You can still stop here and just go on with your life. Focus on what you are doing, while the sensation takes backstage. Maybe you go on with your mind one more step, and decide that you dislike the sensation, the discomfort. Again you can stop here, and most likely it will fade away. If you continue in your mind chatter further, and reinforce this dislike, by talking about it, telling others about it, analyzing it, even getting upset at the dentist or the whole medical system—throwing out claims that the system is corrupt and that's why they gave you this cheap anesthesia—you are adding pain to the basic sensation that was there. You are adding pain to the pain. This mind pain, the pain of pain, is what creates suffering. It is what strengthens the neuron knots in the mind and creates a conditioned reaction that will follow in the future, planting a seed of karma. You have the choice to stop your suffering today. Maybe there will still be pain in your life, but the suffering does not need to remain.

By training your subconscious to be aware of your mind's response, of your automatic actions and conditioned behavior, you can stop the response at an early stage, eliminating the chain of reactions that happen as patterns of conditioning. Once you are released from this cycle of automatic reactions, you are moving into a state of freedom, a place of less suffering, and more awareness. When suffering is gone, bliss is what remains. Practicing awareness in daily life as well as meditation will help you take charge of your life.

Sangha, Your Support Group

Sitting to meditate is a great task; there is always something better to do (or so you'll likely tell yourself). Meditation can be very challenging. If you are new to it, you may feel boredom, agitation, or just the struggle to quiet the mind, which will often call up thoughts we believed were long gone. Sitting alone is wonderful, and in addition, sitting in a group environment can be a good way to enhance the practice. In many of the Buddhist traditions, meditation is done in groups.

Most meditation centers have a variety of offerings, from individual sittings of various lengths, including half-day and even ten-day sits. Some combine the sitting with walking meditation, and some with a talk about the practice.

If you look for a Zen center near you, you will probably find that they have hours when they are open to the public for an intro session. There are also insight meditation centers and Tibetan centers, which may offer slight variations on their techniques of meditation. You can always try and decide for yourself if it is something that resonates with you.

The benefit of a longer practice period is huge. When sitting for a few sessions in a row, the mind begins to tire from repeating the same thoughts, and sometimes it's just easier to drop away. Sometimes the body gets very uncomfortable, and since there is no escaping the sitting, the only way out of suffering is to change the state of mind, dropping the mind's reaction to the pain and going beyond its thoughts of how bad the situation is. Many times the great revelations happen during these longer sitting periods.

Explore and find out what resonates with you and what is convenient for you. The specific group of people—the *sangha*—may be a big part of your decision. If nothing is available in your area, you can create your own sangha by finding a friend or partner who will sit with you at regular times. It may even develop into a small sitting group. Whether you practice alone or in a group, having the support of others can be very helpful.

Review of Sangha: Your Support Group

Find other people that can support your practice. Join yoga classes for yoga asana and meditation groups to enhance your practice. Join a sangha even if you practice with them just once a week. Remember to still keep your personal practice alive alongside your sangha practice.

Mind Maintenance

Have you sat down in meditation over and over to clear your mind, to train it to stay focused and feel that it is not getting much easier? Maybe you notice some change but it is very subtle. Why isn't it easier? I have tried a variety of meditations, visualizations, focusing techniques, Tibetan, Osho, and Zen, and the list goes on. They are all wonderful and do work, but I have constantly needed to go back to them for maintenance, and it wasn't getting any easier.

I kept feeding my mind with tons of input; I read every sign I saw, even when not looking for directions, read all the little advertisements at the side of my Facebook page, listened to NPR so much that I knew every inch of progress of the oil spill, and on and on. How could I ever keep up with cleaning my mind when it was just used to reacting to anything that popped up in front of me?

Think of spring cleaning your closet. When you keep your closet clean and don't collect more than you need, when you give away generously the clothes that no longer serve you, you are constantly aware of what you have in the closet, use what you need, and have a great feeling looking at its contents, as it is organized and well maintained.

The same goes for the mind: if you keep your mind clean, then sitting becomes much more efficient. If you collect info that you do not need, you will keep cluttering the mind, and never get to the place of real peace. Maintain a clear mind throughout your life, clutter less now, so that you will have less cleaning to do later.

Review of Healthy Mind Maintenance

- Turn off the TV when not watching a program you need to see.
- Turn off the radio if you are not really focusing on it.
- Listen to less news.
- Keep your eyes on the road. Don't look at every billboard and advertisement along the way.
- Practice reading information you actually want to get.
- Web control: stay focused on the wave you are surfing; it is easy to get distracted and jump at every wave (advertisement, link, notification) that comes your way.
- Be very selective about your input, and take in less language input.
- And my all-time favorite: Practice seeing without labeling. Look at a flower, a tree, or a cloud, and just see. No need to name what you see. Just see, breathe, and maybe even add a smile!

PART 3

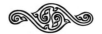

Working with
the Program

By this point you should have a great deal of knowledge, and hopefully some new regular practices. The practices are all great, but what makes the yoga lifestyle so powerful is the combination of these practices into a daily routine. In this final section we will integrate the four components of the flexitarian method—yoga poses, pranayama, food and nutrition, and mind training—into a personalized and sustainable program.

Here you will create a calendar and start building your program. You have some options to choose from, and of course you are welcome to adjust and modify as you need to, but having these programs will make it much more achievable. Once you have the programs, we will look at how to maintain this yoga lifestyle, so that bliss becomes part of you and your life, for now and in the future.

You have come so far along! Be proud of all you've learned and please keep up the good spirit and make these programs happen. Remember, what seems hard at first will flow naturally and with ease over time, like learning to ride a bicycle. So keep the practice alive!

— 8 —

The Flexitarian Method
as a Yoga Lifestyle

Feeling stressed? Having a hard time dealing with all that is coming your way? Life can get overwhelming. There may be many things that need to be taken care of, but most of the time, it is our perception and how we deal with what comes our way that determines if we feel stressed or not.

Tips for Dealing with Stress

Sit and watch. During moments of stress, stop everything, even just for a few seconds, and breathe deeply. Let thoughts appear, observe them, and then go back to what you were doing. Simply being aware of the thoughts as they come and becoming the witness of these thoughts helps us gain a better perspective on what is actually happening.

Do one thing at a time. We often get overwhelmed when there are many things happening at once. Stopping for even a few seconds allows us to connect with the present moment and with that we can tackle the one task that is most crucial. When we are focused on just one thing, all other tasks simply do not exist at that moment, and thus the stress drops away too. In our attempts to get so many things done all at once, we never actually accomplish any of them. Prioritize, and then focus on one thing. Close all alerts so you have fewer distractions and causes of stress.

Practice 1:2 breathing. This helps calm the nervous system and lets the fight-or-flight mechanism subside so you can actually take action from a calm and clear place. You can do just a few rounds whenever you feel a bit overwhelmed or stressed. You can also sit or lie down and practice ten rounds (inhaling to a count of four and exhaling to a count of eight), to really shift your nervous system.

Take a deep breath. Yes, so easy, and yet it does wonders. The main thing is to focus on a long slow exhale. This is really just one round of the 1:2 breathing. For example, suppose you have reached a red light and you are already late. Take a big breath, and slowly release it. Or suppose someone is being slow to pay at the supermarket. You have a meeting to attend, or your kid is screaming—take a deep breath. If you cannot change the situation, stress will not help; it will only make it worse.

Sit on a cloud. Say what? Yes, just for a few moments, imagine sitting on a cloud and looking down at the world. See the bigger picture. See how small you are, and maybe realize that your situation is less dramatic than what you are making of it. At a given moment, when our minds create stories, situations may appear life-threatening, but most of the time the story we create in our mind is far more dramatic than what is actually happening. Really, the stories we tell ourselves can make things worse. Instead of dealing calmly with the situation, when we are stressed, we normally function less effectively and make more errors.

Meditate. This is a regular practice that will help you stay calm and under control. Any of the meditations in the meditation section can be helpful. For stress, sometimes object meditation works best, as for many of us it is easier to focus on an object than to focus on the breath.

Review of Dealing with Stress

- Sit and observe your thoughts.
- Limit your tasks to one at a time.
- Practice 1:2 breathing.
- Take a deep breath and exhale slowly.
- Sit on a cloud and get a real perspective on life.
- Meditate.

How to Make It Happen

Have a visible calendar. Use a calendar as a rough guide to help you get started. You can use your regular calendar and include all your flexitarian practices in it, along with your other important meetings, or use a separate sheet with just your practices (maybe even include colors and images to entice you to look at it—really make it fun). The most important part is that you actually show up to practice! Make sure your calendar is visible to not only you, but also those that need to support you on your journey. If they know your plans in advance, they will be much more likely to support you with your practice.

Set up regular times for practice. If you know that part of your morning routine includes meditation, pranayama (breath work) and yoga poses, then it is easier to follow the routine than would be the case with random practice times.

Use a timer for meditation. Find something easy to use, that you can easily turn on and off, and that has a pleasant enough sound. Most smartphones have timers. Please, use your timer. Using a timer allows you to have peace of mind—you do not need to worry about how much time has passed or how much is left. You can simply sit without needing to peek at the watch. The timer is also like a watchdog. You simply know you will not get up until you hear the timer.

Remember to have your space set up in an inviting way and to have what you need for practice easily accessible. When you need too much time to set up or organize your space for sitting in meditation, pranayama, yoga asana, or even preparing your food, you may find excuses for why you don't have the time or get annoyed with the process. The flexitarian practices for some of us are challenging enough; try to make everything around it easy and welcoming.

Tips for Making Your Practice Happen
- Have a visible calendar, and check it daily.
- Set up regular practice times, remember them, and follow them.
- Use a timer for meditation, so you can be worry free of time.
- Set up your space to be welcoming and easy.

Programs

There are a few programs below. You do not need to follow them, but many times having a set program, even if you are not able to follow it perfectly, is far more efficient than having no program. The 22-day jump-start program is a great place to start, and good for anytime you feel you have dropped off the wagon and need to get back into a routine again. It is also a great place to start again after an injury; just make sure you consult with a professional before you do anything that may incur any risk.

When cardio is mentioned, you can choose anything that feels right for you: swimming, dancing, walking, riding a bike, etc.

If the evenings are not an option (maybe you have kids or some other life affair), consider doing half of what is required. Even five rounds of 1:2 breathing are far better than nothing.

You may need to practice the first week for a while before you move on. Take your time. Get comfortable with what you are practicing before you move on.

Once you have completed this program and you feel like you can maintain it, try to continue practicing days 15–22 regularly. Once you are comfortable with this, move on to the maintenance program.

22-Day Jump-Start Program

Days 1–3
Morning

- Setting intention: 2 minutes
- Yoga asana: 30 minutes
- Ujjayi breath: 5 minutes

Evening

- 1:2 breathing: 10 rounds

Days 4–6
Morning

- Setting intention: 2 minutes
- Yoga asana: 30–45 minutes
- Ujjayi breath: 5 minutes

Evening

- 1:2 breathing: 10 rounds
- Meditation: 5 minutes

Day 7
Morning

- Setting intention: 2 minutes
- Nadi shodhana: 5 rounds
- Viparita karani: 5 minutes
- Meditation: 10 minutes

Days 8, 10, and 12
Morning

- Setting intention: 2 minutes
- Kapalabhati
- Yoga asana: 45–60 minutes
- Meditation: 5–10 minutes

Evening

- 1:2 breathing: 10 rounds
- Meditation: 10 minutes

Days 9, 11, and 13
Morning

- Setting intention: 2 minutes
- Kapalabhati
- Cardio (walk/run/swim/bike): 45 minutes

Evening

- 1:2 breathing: 10 rounds
- Meditation: 10 minutes

Day 14
Morning

- Finding gratitude: 2 minutes

- Nadi shodhana: 5 rounds

- Viparita karani: 5 minutes

- Meditation: 15 minutes

Days 15–21
Morning

- Setting intention: 2 minutes

- Kapalabhati

- Yoga asana: 60–75 minutes

- Meditation: 5–10 minutes

Evening

- 1:2 breathing: 10 rounds

- Meditation: 10–20 minutes

Day 22

- Nadi shodhana: 10 rounds

- Viparita karani: 5 minutes

- Meditation: 20 minutes

Maintenance Program

This is a wonderful intermediate program that is perfect to follow for life. For those new to this practice, it is advised to complete the 22-day jump-start program first. Get comfortable with that and then move on to the maintenance program. You can repeat days 15–22 of the 22-day program for a while until you are comfortable and then move on to the maintenance program.

I offer here a weekly practice that can be continued on a regular basis. You can modify it according to your needs, but this is a good place to start. Both when and for how long you meditate can be modified. Maybe you would rather do it after the pranayama (breath work) practice, as you are already prepared for it, or maybe after the yoga poses, as you have released some energy—either way is fine. Sit for as long as you can: five minutes or thirty minutes. Make sure you decide on your minimum sitting time ahead of time and use a timer. You can always turn the timer off and keep sitting if it feels right. Try to do a longer sit of twenty to forty minutes at least once a week using any type of meditation that resonates with you.

When three-part breathing is offered, you can practice the four-part breathing variation instead.

Fun activities such as walks, hikes, gardening, playing with the kids, or any other physical activity can be added anytime—the more the better.

Days 1, 2, 4, and 6
Morning

- Setting intention: 2 minutes
- Kapalabhati
- Three-part breathing: 5 rounds
- Yoga asana: 60–75 minutes
- Meditation: 10 minutes

Evening

- Meditation: 10 minutes
- 1:2 breathing: 10 rounds

Days 3 and 5
Morning

- Setting intention: 2 minutes
- Nadi shodhana: 5–10 rounds
- Meditation: 10 minutes

Anytime

- Cardio (walk/run/swim/bike): 45 minutes

Evening

- 1:2 breathing: 10 rounds

Day 7

- Rest

- If you like, go for a walk, garden, or anything playful

28-Day Enhancement Program

Are you comfortable with the maintenance program? If so, you may be ready to take it a step further. You may want to do this program every six months or just do it as a one-week enhancement every month or two.

The program is set up as a four-week challenge. You can simply repeat the first week four times, or you can make a few changes, such as adding a longer meditation or pranayama if those are areas you would like to give some extra attention to.

I like to start it on a Sunday to prepare for the week. Monday through Thursday are a bit tougher days; Friday slow down, and Saturday you rest. Of course you can switch it around some to match your schedule.

Day 1
Morning

- Setting intention: 2 minutes

- Viloma pranayama: 6 rounds

- Yoga asana: 60–75 minutes

- Meditation: 15 minutes

Evening

- 1:2 breathing: 10 rounds

- Chant and meditation: 10 minutes

Days 2 and 4
Morning

- Setting intention: 2 minutes

- Kapalabhati: 2 rounds

- Yoga asana: 75–90 minutes

- Nadi shodhana: 5–10 rounds
- Meditation: 5–10 minutes

Evening
- Meditation: 10 minutes
- 1:2 breathing: 10 rounds (lying down)

Days 3 and 5
Morning
- Setting intention: 2 minutes
- Kapalabhati: 1–2 rounds
- Sitali: 2–4 rounds
- Nadi shodhana: 4–8 rounds
- Meditation: 5 minutes
- Cardio: 45 minutes

Evening
- Meditation: 20 minutes

Day 6
Morning
- Setting intention: 2 minutes
- Meditation: 20 minutes
- Kapalabhati: 1–2 rounds
- Sitali: 2–4 rounds
- Nadi shodhana: 4–8 rounds
- Yoga asana: 60–75 minutes

Evening
- Go out; have some fun!

Day 7

Take a break. Do something fun like go to the beach, swim in a lake, go for a walk or a bike ride, etc. If you are craving more yoga, do some yin or restorative yoga.

One-Day Vata Balancing Program

This program is great for everyone but especially for those that feel a bit of vata imbalance (see the Ayurveda chapter). Since vata is the main moving force of our mind, many experience vata imbalance even if it is not their main dosha. I offer a one-day balance, but you can do this a few times a week as needed.

Morning

- Setting intention: 2 minutes
- Kapalbhati: 1–2 rounds
- Viloma pranayama: 6 rounds
- Yoga asana, slow motion with longer held poses: 30 minutes
- Nadi shodhana: 6 rounds
- Chant or object meditation: 10 minutes

Evening

- Chant or mantra: 5 minutes
- Meditation: 10–20 minutes
- 1:2 breathing: 10 rounds (lying down)

These programs bring together the yoga poses practice with the breath work and meditation practices. Keep your food and nutrition part of life in balance, as well, to support these programs. Work with these programs slowly and patiently, but be diligent and actually pursue them. It is better to modify some if needed, than to skip altogether. Remember to show up, that is always the first step. Then keep practicing. In the following chapter I'll give you some tips on how to maintain these practices and states of mind. They work to reinforce these programs.

— 9 —

Maintenance Leads to Bliss

The first step in anything is the hardest. Since you are holding this book, you have already taken that step and hopefully, have begun practicing. Now comes one more challenge: maintaining the practice so your life is sustainable with happiness and health. You may have already figured out how to incorporate all we have learned so far into your life, but here are a few more tips to make it last.

Create a Healthy Environment

The more you set yourself up for success, the more it will happen. You need to set your entire life in a new direction. When shopping for groceries, make sure you only buy the foods that are good for you. Remove foods that are not good for you from your home, so you will not be tempted.

When meeting a friend, consider going for a walk together rather than sitting at a café or a bakery. Even I would not be able to resist a chocolate croissant! This is also true for going to a bar. It's okay to do it sometimes, but what if you meet your friend for a meditation event, a walk, a homemade dinner, or herbal tea? The options are limitless. You may need to introduce your friends to some of your practices and food choices, or you may need to add some new friends who share your practices.

It happens to many yoga students that after they change to the yoga lifestyle, they find a new circle of friends to match this new lifestyle. Since some of their previous friendships may have been all about drinking and going to bars, or other activities that may not fit in their lives anymore, they found new friends that were more aligned with their yoga lifestyle, or "converted" their old friends into the yoga lifestyle too. Now that you wake up earlier, you will need friends that understand your new healthy lifestyle. You may find them at the yoga studio or meditation center. Life is in constant change and so are you. You will have to not only be happy with some new lifestyle changes, but also let go of some old ones that do not serve you.

As much as you can, cook your meals at home, rather than go out to a restaurant. You will be in control of what and how much you eat. Cooking not only lets you choose the ingredients, but you also make the food yourself with your own care and love. The practice of taking care of yourself is important and empowering.

Have your yoga and meditation space ready to go or easy to set up. It should be as easy as possible to roll out your mat or pull out your meditation cushion. Don't give your mind time to find excuses for why it is too much of a hassle to do your practice.

Remember to shut down all possible distractions when you practice—phone, TV, computer, etc. You may even need to tell your family you are going to do your practice, and they will need to learn that this is *your* special time. You can also educate your friends about what you are doing. Maybe they will join you, or at least learn to respect what you need. Surround yourself with positive, supportive, and encouraging people!

When your life and environment are set up, it is more inviting to practice. If you love flowers, place them where you will sit for meditation. If you are disturbed by clutter, straighten up your space before you practice; otherwise when it's time to practice, you will find yourself spending time on creating the space rather than practicing.

Review of Creating a Healthy Environment

- Shop healthy.
- Keep only what is good for you at home.
- Cook your own meals. Invite friends to join.
- Keep your practice area welcoming and ready.
- Make your meetings with friends supportive of your practice.
- Find new friends if needed.
- Educate your family and friends about your new priorities so they can support you.
- Surround yourself with positive, supportive, and encouraging people!

The Positive Box

In Hebrew there is a saying: "Life and death are a matter of the tongue," which means that what you say is as powerful as what you do. Say, "I want to go to yoga," not "I should go to yoga." This will create the right attitude towards what you do. Give a positive attitude to the things that you know will really make you feel better, even if right now they may seem a bit challenging.

When you are doing or experiencing something, even if it does not feel great but you know it is good for you, chose your words from the "positive box." Choose to see the glass half full and use positive adjectives. In almost every situation, it is possible to see the good, and when we state the good with words, we reinforce it. Of course, it is possible to simply be fully present with the experience and not need to describe it at all, but for most of us it is too hard to be fully mindful and present; thus it is better to choose from the positive box until you get to the point where you simply *are*.

Our minds are very powerful, and our speech and thoughts are manifestations of our minds, as well as reinforcements to what is already there. So when you speak in a certain way, you are reinforcing that same attitude. Just by choosing to say things differently, you can create change in your mind and change the way you feel.

A classic example is a long-held yoga pose such as hanuman asana (splits pose). Most people are fine in this pose for a few moments. Then the mind comes rushing in with stories. At times I could hear my mind say, "This is probably enough," or "How do I know I am not getting injured? This is intense!" Or it might say, "Did three minutes already pass? This hurts!"

My practice is to go back to the breath and even add a soft smile. If my mind wants to be active, I breathe in a sense of gratitude that my hamstrings are opening—gratitude that they are stiff from all the hard work they went through, such as running, biking, and much more. I feel the gratitude, the soft smile, and the calm breath. I can even say out loud, "Thank you; this is exactly what I need."

Review of Reinforcing the Good

- Find the good in every situation.
- State what you need positively.
- Use the breath as a neutralizer when needed.
- Find gratitude for something when all else feels bad.
- Practice letting go of the descriptions altogether over time.

Yoga Master Reminders

Sense reminders are powerful. Just like seeing a certain food makes us want it, or smelling something can create a craving, seeing something symbolic of where you want to be can be helpful. Two powerful reminders are notes and symbolic objects.

A note may simply be straightforward. You can make a list of what you are practicing, use a calendar, or just write a few sentences that are your current intentions. Put it somewhere where you see it all the time, like your fridge or bathroom mirror. You can even use a bunch of sticky notes with simple intentions put up in strategic locations. For example, on your computer: "Take a deep breath before starting to work." On the fridge: "Enjoy your greens!" On your dashboard: "Smile with every red light." On your bathroom mirror: "Stay present." On your alarm clock: "Smile."

A symbolic object can simply be a photo of a calm person like a Buddha, a saint, a mermaid, or even a photo of serene nature to remind you of the state of mind you want to be in. It can be a fresh flower placed on your worktable to remind you of your attitude for the day.

The important thing is that you surround yourself with support. Sometimes it will come from other people, and sometimes it will simply be happy reminders to yourself of what you need to do or the attitude you need to have.

Review of the Support System

- Put your practice calendar on the fridge or somewhere visible.
- Place sticky note reminders in strategic locations.
- Place a symbolic reminder of your ideal attitude where you work.
- Ask friends and family to check in on you.
- Place uplifting images or symbolic objects around your home and workplace.

Don't Stress About It

It is easy to get anxious about all you have to do. The more anxious you get and the more you think about what you have to do, the more you create an expectation and fear of not being able to get it done. Once you have an expectation that cannot be met, you are setting yourself up for disappointment and possibly guilt.

The more regular you become with your practice, the easier it gets to just keep it going. If you do find that you have skipped a day of practice or you had an extra brownie at your friend's house or your yoga practice was only thirty minutes for the past three days, it is better to set an intention to adjust what you can from now on, than to beat yourself up for not doing or acting the way you think you should have. When you feel badly about the way you are, you are planting a negative imprint in your mind. This creates a pattern, a seed that will become a rotten fruit.

Look at what is or was, decide how you can improve the situation, and just do it. Simply take the action needed to make the change. We do need to recognize what works for us, and what doesn't, but we do not need to become the angry schoolmaster that punishes the bad student. Practice with delight and joy, knowing that this is good for you!

Review on How to Be Anxiety Free

- Be present. Focus on what is in front of you right now.
- Make a list and prioritize it. Then do the top priority item on the list.
- Reassign whatever you did not manage to finish, and forget about it for now.
- Learn from mistakes and then move on. Don't reassess.
- Be compassionate towards yourself but not lazy.
- Practice with delight.

Being Content: Encouragement

We already spoke about doing the best that you can and being okay with where you are. This is one of the key elements of happiness and total health. There is so much you CAN do, so much you know, so much you have. Remember not to compare yourself to others or even to how you were in the past, but rather be happy about all that you have now.

Keep practicing gratitude, and maybe add some daily practices of self-thanking. Thank yourself every time you do something that is good for you. Thank you, Doron, for eating a salad. Thank you for not choosing the ice cream. Thanks for resisting TV and doing pranayama instead. Thank you for going to sleep a bit earlier—now I can get up early enough to do my yoga practice. Keep encouraging yourself to do the right thing, and give yourself hugs for what you do.

Some people appreciate hugs, while others appreciate a visual sense of accomplishment. You can have your yoga master calendar on the fridge and mark a nice star next to each practice completed. This is a great way to keep you on track.

Review of Self-Encouragement

- Acknowledge your good actions.
- Mark your good actions on your calendar (a gold star sticker, or bright yellow highlight).
- Reward yourself with a healthy treat.
- Share your success with others.

Collaboration

It is not always easy to get motivated to practice or to eat healthy food. Most of us find it easier to dress nicely, behave in proper ways, or try harder with our physical practice if someone else is present. Whether we care about what others think or not, we feel a bit of a need to demonstrate the "right" way of living, or we are simply more committed when someone else is involved.

Find a friend or a partner that will join you in some of the activities—a regular yoga buddy or a healthy lunch friend, for example. You can have a meditation group or just another friend that meets with you twice a week, and during those times practice for thirty or forty minutes instead of the fifteen minutes you do on your own. Zen monasteries live on the concept of sangha, a group of like-minded people that become like a family in sharing their practices.

Choose your friends wisely. See if you can find someone that is at least as committed as you, maybe even more—a good friend for walking or other friends for playing group sports. This is why people go to yoga classes, meet friends for hikes, and join meditation groups. We are social beings, and most of us will do more when in a social environment.

Review of Collaborating Tips

- Have a practice buddy.
- Try to find someone at least as committed as you are.
- Join a meditation group.
- Take yoga classes, and make friends with your yoga buddies.
- Do group sports.

It is easy to start projects, take on a diet, buy a new book, or talk about our intention. But maintaining the initial effort is not as easy. Make sure you do create a healthy environment, have a support system, collaborate with others, and especially be content with what you are doing, and don't stress about it. The yoga lifestyle is realistic and possible, but you need to keep giving it the love and attention it deserves, it will be worth your while.

Conclusion

I have been asking questions about existence since I was a kid. I have always tried not to take things for granted. Old truths inspired me, but I kept challenging them. What is right for me today, in this day and age?

I was twenty-one when I traveled through Asia, searching. I went to every teacher and center that seemed to have answers. I really wanted something more out of life, but I am not even sure I knew what I was looking for. I tasted many different paths and learned about many practices that would help me find peace, happiness, and good health. My search continued in the West: countless schools, friends, classes, and so much reading.

I found that the basic truths have always remained true. Almost all of what I wrote here has not changed over the years. It is only small bits of information that change, mostly related to food, though no one ever contradicted the idea that eating vegetables is good for you.

I do hope that while you practice the teachings I have presented in this book, you stay informed about new research and never take anything for granted. I will keep updating my new findings and personal experiences on my site: www.doronyoga.com.

Now that you have my recipe for a happy, healthy life—for the yoga lifestyle—I hope you find it as transformative as it has been for me. You will notice some changes right away and some over time.

Remember that staying happy is mostly about your attitude, so keep calm and yoga on!

With deep love and gratitude,
Doron

Further Reading

Yoga Asana and Philosophy

Cope, Stephen. *The Wisdom of Yoga: A Seeker's Guide to Extraordinary Living.* New York: Bantam Dell, 2006.

Desikachar, T. K. V. *The Heart of Yoga*: *Developing a Personal Practice.* Rochester, VT: Inner Traditions, 1995.

Iyengar, B. K. S. *Light on Yoga.* New York: Schockten, 1966.

Saraswati, Swami Satyanada. *Four Chapters on Freedom.* Munger, Bihar, India: Publications Trust, 1976.

Stephens, Mark. *Teaching Yoga: Essential Foundations and Techniques.* Berkeley, CA: North Atlantic Books, 2010.

Swenson, David. *Ashtanga Yoga, The Practice Manual: An Illustrated Guide to Personal Practice.* Austin, TX: Ashtanga Yoga Productions, 1999.

Food and Nutrition

Balch, Phyllis, A. *Prescription for Nutritional Healing.* New York: Avery, 2006.
Chopra, Deepak. *Perfect Health.* New York: Three Rivers Press, 2000.

Eisenstein, Charles. *The Yoga of Eating: Transcending Diets and Dogma to Nourish the Natural Self.* Washington, DC: Newtrends Publishing, Inc., 2003.

Frawley, David. *Yoga and Ayurveda: Self-Healing and Self-Realization*. Twin Lakes, WI: Lotus Press, 1999.

Holdford, Patrick. *The New Optimum Nutrition Bible*. Berkeley, CA: The Crossing Press, 2004.

Pitchford, Paul. *Healing with Whole Foods: Asian Traditions and Modern Nutrition*. Berkeley, CA: North Atlantic Books, 1993, 1996, 2002.

Mind Training

Narayan, R. K. *The Guide*. London, England: Penguin Books, 2006.

Suzuki, Shunryu. *Zen Mind, Beginner's Mind*. Boston: Shambhala Publications, 2011.

Tolle, Ekhart. *A New Earth*. New York: Penguin Group, 2005.

———. *The Power of Now*. Novato, CA: New World Library, 1999.

Suggested Films for Education and Inspiration
FOOD AND HEALTH

Forks Over Knives

Food, Inc.

Ingredients

Farmageddon

King Corn

The Future of Food

MIND AND SPIRIT

Project Happiness

Glossary of Asana (Yoga Pose) Names

SANSKRIT NAME	ENGLISH TRANSLATION
Adho Mukha Svanasana	Downward Facing Dog
Adho Mukha Vrksasana	Handstand
Agnistambhasana	Fire Log Pose
Akarna Dhanurasana	Archer's Pose
Anjali Mudra	Salutation Seal
Anjaneyasana	Lunge
Apanasana	Knees to chest pose
Ardha Baddha Padma Paschimottanasana	Half lotus bound seated forward fold
Ardha Baddha Padmottanasana	Half lotus bound standing forward fold
Ardha Chandrasana	Half-Moon Pose
Ardha Matsyendrasana	Half Lord of the Fish Pose
Ashtanga Pranam	Eight Limbed Pose (knees chest chin)
Astavakrasana	Eight Crook's Pose
Baddha Hasta Sirsasana A B C D	Bound Hands Headstand Posture
Baddha Konasana A B	Bound Angle Pose

Baddha Padmasana	Bound Lotus Posture
Bakasana	Crane Pose
Balasana	Child's Pose
Bharadvajasana	Bharadvaja's Twist
Bhekasana	Frog Pose
Bhujangasana	Cobra
Bhujapidasana	Shoulder Squeezing Pose
Bidalasana	Cat pose
Cakrasana	Wheel pose
Chaturanga Dandasana	Four-limbed staff pose
Dandasana	Staff pose
Dhanurasana	Bow pose
Dwi Pada Koundinyasana	Pose of the sage Koundinya
Dwi Pada Viparita Dandasana	Both feet inverted staff pose
Eka Pada Bakasana	One-legged crane pose
Eka Pada Koundinyasana	Pose dedicated to the sage Koundinya
Eka Pada Rajakapotasana	One-legged king pigeon pose
Eka Pada Sirsasana A B C	One foot behind head pose
Eka Pada Viparita Dandasana	One-footed inverted staff pose
Galavasana	Pose dedicated to the sage Galava
Garbha Pindasana	Embryo pose
Garudasana	Eagle pose
Gomukhasana A B	Cow pace pose
Halasana	Plow pose

Hanumanasana	Monkey pose (splits)
Janu Sirsasana	Head-to-knee forward bend
Jathara Parivartanasana	Belly twisting pose
Kapotasana	Pigeon pose
Karandavasana	Duck posture
Kasyapasana	Pose dedicated to the sage Kasyapa
Karnapidasana	Ear pressure posture
Krounchasana	Heron pose
Kukkutasana	Rooster pose
Kurmasana	Tortoise pose
Laghu Vajrasana	Little thunderbolt pose
Lolasana	Dangling earring pose
Maha Mudra	Great seal
Malasana	Garland pose (squat)
Marichyasana A B C D	Pose dedicated to the sage Marichi
Matsyasana	Fish pose
Mayurasana	Peacock pose
Mukta Hasta Sirsana	Hands free headstand pose
Nakrasana	Crocodile pose
Natarajasana	Lord of the Dance pose
Navasana	Boat pose
Padangusthasana	Toe lifting standing pose
Padahastasana	Foot hand standing pose
Padmasana	Lotus pose

Parighasana	Gate pose
Parivrtta Ardha Chandrasana	Revolved half-moon pose
Parivrtta Janu Sirsasana	Revolved head to knee pose
Parivrtta Parsvakonasana	Revolved side angle pose
Parivrtta Trikonasana	Revolved triangle pose
Parivrtta Utkatasana	Revolved (awkward) chair pose
Parsva bakasana	Sideways crane pose
Parsvottanasana	Intense side stretch pose
Parsva Dhanurasana	Side bow
Pashasana	Noose pose
Paschimottanasana	Seated forward bend
Pincha Mayurasana	Feathered peacock pose
Pindasana	Embryo pose
Prasarita Padottanasana A B C D	Intense spread-legged stretch
Purvottanasana	Upward facing/Eastern intense stretch pose
Shalabhasana A B	Locust pose
Salamba Sarvangasana	Supported shoulder stand
Salamba Sirsasana	Supported headstand
Samasthiti	Equanimous place pose
Savasana	Corpse pose
Salamba Setu Bandhasana	Bridge pose
Simhasana	Lion Pose
Sirsasana A B	Headstand
Setu Bandhasana	Bridge pose

Sukhasana	Easy/Happy pose
Supta Baddha Konasana	Reclining bound angle pose
Supta Konasana	Reclining angle pose
Supta Kurmasana	Reclining Tortoise Pose
Supta Padangusthasana	Reclining big toe pose
Supta Urdhva Pada Vajrasana	Reclining raised foot thunderbolt pose
Supta Vajrasana	Reclining thunderbolt pose
Supta Virasana	Reclining hero pose
Tadasana	Mountain pose
Trianga Mukha Eka Pada Paschimottanasana	One foot facing up forward bend
Tittibhasana A B C D	Insect pose
Tolasana	Scale pose
Ubhaya Padangusthasana A B C	Upright hand to big toe pose
Upavishta Konasana A B	Seated wide angle pose
Urdhva Dhanurasana	Upward facing bow
Urdhva Hastasana	Hands over head pose
Urdhva Mukha Paschimottanasana	Upward facing/Western intense stretch pose
Urdhva Padmasana	Upward lotus pose
Urdhva Prasarita Eka Padasana	Standing split
Ustrasana	Camel pose
Utkatasana	Fierce Pose
Uttana Padasana	Extended leg pose
Uttanasana	Standing forward fold

Utthita Hasta Padangusthasana	Extended hand big toe pose
Utthita Parsvakonasana	Extended side angle pose
Utthita Trikonasana	Extended triangle pose
Vasisthasana	Pose of Vaishista
Vatayanasana	Horse pose
Viparita dandasana	Inverted staff pose
Virabhadrasana I, II, III	Warrior 1, 2, and 3
Vrksasana	Tree pose
Vrishchikasana	Scorpion pose
Yoganidrasana	Yogi's sleep pose

Glossary of Yoga, Meditation, and Pranayama Terminology

Acharya: a respectful add-on to a name, an instructor or guru. For example, Krishnamacharya

Adho: downward

Adho Mukha: downward facing

Agni: fire

Ahimsa: non-harming; one of the Yamas, a sub group of the eight limbs of Patanjali, and an important moral discipline of non-violence

Anjali Mudra: the gesture of Anjali, hands together in front of the heart

Ananda: bliss; the state one realizes when in Samadhi, or the realization of true and ultimate reality

Anga: limb; used mostly to describe one of the foundations of Patanjali's system of Ashtanga or the eight limbs

Apana: the downward energy towards the pelvis or lower abdomen; the energy responsible for the elimination of waste products from the body

Ardha: half

Asana: seat; the third limb in Patanjali's Ashtanga Yoga, a physical posture meant for meditation. The term later became used to describe a variety of poses, such as in the Hatha Yoga Pradipika, and today it is used to describe the physical practice of yoga.

Ashram: a spiritual home, a hermitage, a place where one practices

Ashtanga yoga: eight-limbed union; Patanjali's system described in eight parts, or limbs. Ashtanga consists of moral discipline (yama), self-restraint (niyama), posture (asana), breath control (pranayama), sensory control (pratyahara), concentration (dharana), meditation (dhyana), and bliss (samadhi).

Awareness: consciousness of all that is in the present moment

Ayurveda: the science of life; India's traditional medicine system, a system that looks at the root cause of the problem rather than the symptoms

Baka: crane

Bandha: a bond or a lock. In yoga these are like control centers). There are three main bandhas are mula bandha, uddiyana bandha, and jalandhara bandha. These control centers are one of the three pillars of Ashtanga Yoga described by Krishnamacharya; the bandhas generate physical and energetic reactions.

Bhujanga: cobra

Buddha: the awakened one; one who has attained enlightenment; also the name for Gautama, the founder of Buddhism, who lived in the sixth century B.C.E.

Chandra: moon

Danda: staff or stick

Danu: bow

Dharma: path, teachings, universal law. Dharma is one of the three pillars of Buddhism and has a variety of meanings, such as the path, the teaching, or the law. We study the dharma, follow the dharma, and obey the dharma, or we can be people of dharma (of virtue).

Dristi: view, gaze; one of three pillars of Ashtanga as described by Krishnamacharya; there are a variety of points on which the dristi is focused, such as at the tip of the nose or the spot between the eyebrows, to help in focus, concentration, and deepening of the pose.

Dwi: two

Eka: one

Eka Pada: one-legged, or one-footed

Garuda: eagle; the king of birds; having a white face, red wings, and a golden body, Garuda serves as Vishnu's vehicle.

Gayatri mantra: a famous Vedic mantra often recited at sunrise: om bhur bhu vat svaha, tat savitur varenyam bhargo devasya dhimahi dhiyo yo nah pracodayat

Gomukha: cow head

Guru: a spiritual teacher. The one who shows the light.

Hala: plough

Hatha Yoga: forceful yoga; a major branch of yoga developed by Goraksha and other adepts c. 1000 C.E. that emphasizes the physical aspects of the transformative path, notably postures (asana), cleansing techniques (shodhana), and breath control (pranayama).

Hanuman: a monkey God, son of Anjneya and Vayu

Hasta: hand or arm

Ida Nadi: the left side energy channel that leads prana up from the base chakra. Ida nadi is associated with the parasympathetic nervous system and has a cooling or calming effect on the mind when activated.

Janu: knee

Jathara: belly

Karma: action, often thought of as the consequences of one's own actions

Karma Yoga: yoga of action based on the teachings of the Bhagavad Gita; Krishna teaches action according to one's duty without self-consideration.

Kapala: skull

Kapha: one of the three Ayurvedic humors

Kapota: pigeon

Karna: ear

Kona: angle

Krama: a sequence or succession of moments

Kumbhaka: breath retention used in pranayama (breath work)

Lola: to swing or dangle

Mala: garland, wreath

Manduka: frog

Matsyendra: Lord of Fish. Matsyendra is an early tantric master who founded the Yogini Kaula School and is remembered as a teacher of Goraksha.

Mudra: seal; a spiritual gesture, mostly done with hands and fingers, though there are some whole-body mudras. In yoga, mudras are used together with pranayama (breath work) to control the flow of prana (life force) in the body.

Mukha: face

Mula: root, base

Mula Bandha: root lock; root control center, the lifting of the perineum and activation of the PC muscle, creating an energetic stimulation

Nadi: conduit; one of the 72,000 or more subtle channels along or through which the life force (prana) circulates; the three most important are the ida nadi, pingala nadi, and sushumna nadi

Nadi shodhana: a pranayama (breath work) practice intended to cleanse and purify the channels of energy in the body

Namaskara: salutation, greeting

Nataraja: Dancing Shiva

Nauli: physical purification, a technique of churning the belly

Nidra: sleep, relaxation

Nirvana: ultimate attainment

Om: sometimes spelled ohm or aum; consisting of three sounds—A, U, and M, it is the original mantra symbolizing the ultimate reality and is a prefix to many mantric utterances

Parivrtta: crossed, with a twist

Parsva: side, lateral

Patanjali: compiler of the Yoga Sutra who lived c. 150 C.E.

Pingala Nadi: the right side energy channel that leads prana up from the base chakra. It's associated with the sympathetic nervous system and has an energizing effect on the mind when activated.

Pitta: one of the three Ayurvedic humors

Prajna: wisdom; a tool for liberation in Buddhism, the others being skillful means (upaya) and compassion (karuna)

Prakriti: nature on all its levels, from physical to energetic. It is the changeable or observed, in contrast to purusha (the supreme consciousness). Prakriti is composed of three essential characteristics (gunas): sattva, rajas, and tamas.

Prana: life, breath; the life force that sustains the body; the breath as an external manifestation of the subtle life force

Pranayama: the extension of life force through breath control practices. In this manual we call it breath work.

Pratikriyasana: counter pose

Pratyahara: withdrawal; sensory inhibition; the fifth limb (anga) of Patanjali's Ashtanga yoga

Puraka: inhalation used in pranayama (breath work)

Purna: complete, infinite

Purusha: the transcendental self (atman) or spirit, a designation that is mostly used in samkhya and Patanjali's yoga to differentiate from prakriti (nature). Purusha is unchangeable.

Raja: king, ruler

Raja Yoga: Royal Yoga; a late medieval designation of Patanjali's ashtanga yoga, also known as classical yoga

Rechaka: exhalation used in pranayama (breath work)

Sadhana: spiritual discipline leading to siddhi (perfection or accomplishment); the term is specifically used in tantra

Sama: equal, same

Samadhi: putting together; the state in which the consciousness of the meditator is unified with the object of meditation; the eighth and final limb (anga) of Patanjali's ashtanga yoga.

Sangha: spiritual community or those who practice according to the Dharma taught by Buddha

Santosha: contentment; one of the niyamas of Patanjali's ashtanga yoga

Sat: pure, true essence, universal spirit, truth

Shodhana: cleansing, purifying; one of the foundations of all yoga paths is to purify

Sitali: a cooling form of pranayama (breath work)

Stirha: steady, controlled, firm

Sukha: ease, happiness

Sushmna-nadi: the main nadi (energy channel) through which kundalini shakti (kundalini power) rises.

Supta: supine, sleeping

Surya: sun

Sutra: thread; an aphoristic statement

Svana: dog

Tamas: inertia, heaviness, sluggishness, obstruction, sloth; resistance to action; one of the three gunas

Tri: three

Uddiyana: upward flying

Uddiyana bandha: flying up, a lock or control center. An action of drawing the lower abdominal core in and up.

Ujjayi: victorious

Utpluti: pumping or lifting up

Utthita: extended

Vatta: one of the three Ayurvedic humors

Vinyasa: to place in a specific way, or in today's terms, the conscious connection of breath and movement

Vipassana: insight, seeing clearly; the direct perception (not thinking about or verbalizing) of the true nature of things. There is no vipassana technique per se, only techniques such as anapanasati (mindfulness of breath), which prepare the mind for vipassana.

Vriksha: tree

Yoga: union; from the root yuj, meaning to yoke or to make whole

Zen: a Buddhist school from the Mahayana tradition. Emphasis is placed on the practice of Zazen and the work with a spiritual teacher, to get direct experience and understand the true self (Buddha nature). Zen emphasizes the daily practice as a practice for the benefit of others.

Bibliography and Resources

Appleton, Nancy. *Lick The Sugar Habit.* 2nd Edition. New York: Avery, 1988.

Balch, Phyllis, A. *Prescription for Nutritional Healing.* New York: Avery, 2006.

Bhagavad Gita, The Song of the Lord. Trans. Swami Prabhavananda and Christopher Isherwood. New York: Signet Classic, 2002.

Buddhananada, Swami. *Moola Bandha: The Master Key.* Munger, Bihar, India: Yoga Publications Trust, 1978, 1996.

Chopra, Deepak. *Perfect Health.* New York: Three Rivers Press, 2000.

Colbin, Annemarie. *Food and Healing: How What You Eat Determines Your Health, Your Well-Being, and the Quality of Your Life.* New York: Ballantine Books, 1986.

Cope, Stephen. *The Wisdom of Yoga: A Seeker's Guide to Extraordinary Living.* New York: Bantam Dell, 2006.

Desikachar, T. K. V. *The Heart of Yoga: Developing a Personal Practice.* Rochester, VT: Inner Traditions, 1995.

Dimon, Theodore, Jr. *Anatomy of the Moving Body: A Basic Course in Bones, Muscles, and Joints.* Berkeley, CA: North Atlantic Books, 2001, 2008.

Dreyer, Danny. *Chi Running.* New York: Fireside, 2009.

Eisenstein, Charles. *The Yoga of Eating: Transcending Diets and Dogma to Nourish the Natural Self.* Washington, DC: Newtrends Publishing, Inc., 2003.

Feuerstein, Georg. *Yoga Tradition: Its History, Literature, Philosophy, and Practice.* Prescott, AZ: Hohm Press, 1998, 2001, 2008.

Frawley, David. *Yoga and Ayurveda: Self-Healing and Self-Realization.* Twin Lakes, WI: Lotus Press, 1999.

Freeman, Richard. *The Mirror of Yoga: Awakening the Intelligence of Body and Mind.* Boston, MA: Shambhala, 2010.

Goldstein, Joseph, and Jack Kornfield. *Seeking the Heart of Wisdom: The Path of Insight Meditation.* Boston, MA: Shambhala, 1987.

Greene, Joshua, M. *Gita Wisdom*: *An Introduction to India's Essential Yoga Text.* San Rafael, CA: Mandala, 2008.

Hanh, Thich Nhat. *Anger: Wisdom for Cooling the Flames.* New York: Riverhead Books, 2001.

Holdford, Patrick. *The New Optimum Nutrition Bible.* Berkeley, CA: The Crossing Press, 2004.

Huber, Cheri. *Suffering is Optional: Three Keys to Freedom and Joy.* Keep It Simple Books, 2000.

Iyengar, B. K. S. *Light on Pranayama*: *The Yogic Art of Breathing.* New York: Crossroad, 1985.

———. *Light on Yoga.* New York: Schockten, 1966.

———. *Light on the Yoga Sutras of Patanjali.* Columbia, MO: South Asia, 1993.

Judith, Anodea. *Eastern Body Western Mind: Psychology and the Chakra System as a Path to the Self.* Berkeley, CA: Celestial Arts, 1996, 2004.

Kaminoff, Leslie, and Amy Matthews. *Yoga Anatomy: Your Illustrated Guide to Postures, Movements, and Breathing Techniques.* Champaign, IL: Human Kinetics, 2012, 2007.

Krishnamurti, J. *On Relationship*. Hampshire, England: Krishnamurti Foundation India, 1992.

———. *Total Freedom: The Essential Krishnamurti*. Hampshire, England: Krishnamurti Foundation Trust Ltd., 1996.

Long, Ray. *The Key Muscles of Yoga: Your Guide to Functional Anatomy in Yoga*. Bandha Yoga, 2005, 2006.

———. *The Key Poses of Yoga: Your Guide to Functional Anatomy in Yoga*. Bandha Yoga, 2008.

Loori, John Daido. *Sitting with Koans: The Essential Writings on the Practice of Zen Koan Introspection*. Somerville, MA: Wisdom Publications, 2006.

Maehle, Gregor. *Ashtanga Yoga: Practice and Philosophy*. Novato, CA: New World Library, 2006.

McGee, Harold. *On Food and Cooking: The Science and Lore of the Kitchen*. New York: Scribner, 1984, 2004.

Muktibodhananda, Swami. *Swara Yoga: The Tantric Science of Brain Breathing*. Munger, Bihar, India: Yoga Publications Trust, 1984.

Murray, Michael. *Encyclopedia of Healing Foods*. New York: Atria Books, 2005.

Narayan, R. K. *The Guide*. London: Penguin Books, 2006.

Osho. *The Alchemy of Yoga*: *Commentaries on the Yoga Sutras of Patanjali*. Pune, MS, India: Tao Publishing, 1977.

———. *The Book of Man*. New Delhi, India: Penguin Books, 2002, 2004.

———. *The Book of Nothing*. Pune, MS, India: Tao Publishing, 1975.

———. *The Essence of Yoga*. New Delhi, India: Penguin Books, 2003.

———. *The Path of Yoga: Talks on the Yoga Sutras of Patanjali*. Pune, MS. India: Rebel, 1973, 2008.

Pitchford, Paul. *Healing with Whole Foods: Asian Traditions and Modern Nutrition.* Berkeley, CA: North Atlantic Books, 1993, 1996, 2002.

Prabhavananda, Swami. *Patanjali Yoga Sutras.* Mylapore, Chennai: Sri Ramakrishna Math Printing Press.

Radhakrishan, S. *The Principle Upanishads.* New Delhi, India: Harper Collins Publishers, 2007.

Saraswati, Swami, Satyananda. *Four Chapters on Freedom.* Munger, Bihar, India: Yoga Publications Trust, 1976.

———. *Kundalini Tantra.* Munger, Bihar, India: Yoga Publications Trust, 1984.

———. *Taming the Kundalini.* Mungar, Bihar, India: Yoga Publications Trust, 1967.

Schiffmann, Eric. *Yoga: The Spirit and Practice of Moving into Stillness.* New York: Pocket Books, 1996.

Scott, John. *Ashtanga Yoga: The Definitive Step-by-Step Guide to Dynamic Yoga.* New York: Three Rivers Press, 2000.

Singleton, Mark. *Yoga Body: The Origins of Modern Posture Practice.* New York: Oxford University Press, 2010.

Stephens, Mark. *Teaching Yoga: Essential Foundations and Techniques.* Berkeley, CA: North Atlantic Books, 2010.

Suzuki, Shunryu. *Zen Mind, Beginner's Mind.* Boston, MA: Shambhala Publications, 2011.

Svatmarama. *The Hatha Yoga Pradipika.* Trans. Brian Dana Akers. Woodstock, NY: YogaVidya, 2002.

Svoboda, Robert, E. *Prakriti: Your Ayurvedic Constitution.* Delhi, India: Motilal Banarsidass Publishers, 2005.

Swenson, David. *Ashtanga Yoga, The Practice Manual: An Illustrated Guide to Personal Practice.* Austin, TX: Ashtanga Yoga Productions, 1999.

Thomas, Benjamin, A., and Tommijean Thomas. *Astanga Yoga: In the Iyengar Tradition.* 2004.

Tolle, Ekhart. *A New Earth.* New York: Penguin Group, 2005.

———. *The Power of Now.* Novato, CA: New World Library, 1999.

Watts, Alan. *Does it Matter: Essays on Man's Relation to Materiality.* Novato, CA: New World Library, 2007.

———. *The Way of Zen.* New York: Vintage Books, 1957.

White, Ganga. *Yoga Beyond Belief: Insights to Awaken and Deepen Your Practice.* Berkeley, CA: North Atlantic Books, 2007.

Wolfe, Jennifer. *Prenatal Vinyasa Yoga Manual: A Guide to Safely Integrating Pregnant Women into your Vinyasa Classes.* 2012.

Wood, Rebecca. *The New Whole Foods Encyclopedia.* New York: Penguin Books, 2010.

Vivekananda, Swami. *Jnana Yoga: The Yoga of Knowledge.* Kolkata, India: Advaita Ashram, 2004.

About the Author

Doron is a lifelong student of meditation, yoga, health, and nutrition. After dabbling in some psychology, Doron went on a two-year study/travel exploration through Asia. He stayed at Osho's ashram, studied yoga in Rishikesh, studied with the Dalai Lama, practiced Vipassana in Thailand, lived and worked with a Buddhist priest in Japan, and, most of all, learned from his own experiences. He traveled in India as locals do, slept in the most basic places, lived the "middle way" in Thailand, tried luxury in Japan, and through it all met amazing people who were all teachers in their own way.

The spark for understanding the world, himself, and the meaning of happiness never left Doron, and he continued to devote time and effort to studying and practicing meditation, yoga, cooking, and a variety of healing modalities, such as Reiki, massage, energy work, and dance. He worked at the best raw food restaurant in North America—Pure Foods and Wine—and later completed a culinary residency at the prestigious Montalvo art resident program, where he founded a sustainable garden, taught nutrition to kids, and started a yoga program for the staff and residents.

Next, he spent a year at Esalen as a student of Gestalt, dance, and community living. While there, he worked in the kitchen as a chef and taught workshops about yoga and nutrition.

Doron has taken countless workshops and classes, and has been on countless health and meditation retreats at ashrams, Tibetan centers, and Zen centers. He returns to India regularly to deepen his yoga and Ayurveda studies, take cooking classes, and study yoga philosophy.

Doron is a yoga instructor certified by the Yoga Alliance (ERYT 500), a certified nutrition consultant, a certified holistic chef, and a member of the American Society of Drugless Practitioners. He published a poetry book in Hebrew titled *Now I Am Here*, which brought forth his continuous quest for harmony between his inner truth and the life he felt he needed to live.

To Write to the Author

If you wish to contact the author or would like more information about this book, please write to the author in care of Llewellyn Worldwide, Ltd. and we will forward your request. The authors and publisher appreciate hearing from you and learning of your enjoyment of this book and how it has helped you. Llewellyn Worldwide, Ltd. cannot guarantee that every letter written to the author can be answered, but all will be forwarded. Please write to:

Doron Hanoch
℅ Llewellyn Worldwide
2143 Wooddale Drive
Woodbury, MN 55125-2989

Please enclose a self-addressed stamped envelope for reply, or $1.00 to cover costs.
If outside the USA, enclose an international postal reply coupon.